Living Well

With Kidney Disease

Living Well

With Kidney Disease

FIRST EDITION

A RESOURCE FOR PATIENTS AND THEIR FAMILIES

Based on the handbook,
When Your Kidneys Fail
By Mickie Hall Faris, MPH, MBA,
1982

Editor Elaine S. Kamil, MD
Assistant Editor Katherine Bolden, RN, MSN

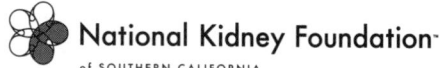 **National Kidney Foundation**
of SOUTHERN CALIFORNIA
17100 Ventura Blvd., Suite 222
Encino, CA 91316
800.747.5527
www.kidneysocal.org

Published and Distributed by the
National Kidney Foundation
of Southern California (NKFSC)
17100 Ventura Blvd. Suite 222
Encino, CA 91316
800.747.5527
www.kidneysocal.org

Living Well With Kidney Disease
Copyright 2007 by the
National Kidney Foundation
Of Southern California

Editor Elaine S. Kamil, MD
Assistant Editor Katherine Bolden, RN, MSN
Managing Editor Ann M. Giblin

Library of Congress Catalogue Card Number: TXU 1-319-715

Printed in the United States of America
Cover design, Jennifer Hocutt

To all people

living with chronic kidney failure,

who asked the questions

and inspired us to search

for the answers.

Foreword

I encountered the pioneering stages of dialysis therapy, beginning in 1968 at age two. Following 12 years on dialysis (both peritoneal dialysis and hemodialysis) and three kidney transplants—the last of which took place in 1990—I have learned that knowledge coupled with a dose of hope is the key to living a joyful life in spite of chronic kidney disease. I understand the gamut of emotions that come with being diagnosed with chronic illness: the fear, anger, and depression that lead to understanding and acceptance.

If you take an active role in your care, learn all you can, and talk to fellow patients, you can still achieve your dreams and goals.

As a young girl on dialysis, I dreamt of being happily married, having a successful business, and becoming an author. Today at age 39, I can say I have accomplished my dreams and continue to build new ones each day.

You must become your own advocate, ask questions, and adhere to your medical regimen. It is imperative that you learn as much as you can about your illness, reach out to the renal community, find supportive organizations, and get involved.

One such organization that has stood the test of time is the NKF of Southern California. In an area as vast as Southern California, it is easy to lose sight of where the borders of the renal community start and stop. It is only through the efforts of organizations such as the NKFSC that the patients, their families, and the healthcare professionals who make up this community can come together on common ground, reminding us in the process that we're all after the same pursuit—health! I would encourage everyone reading this book to foster that sense of community in their local areas.

Many of these knowledgeable healthcare professionals and patients have provided wonderful educational information in this book that will help you navigate your illness and make choices that are right for you.

Lori Hartwell

Preface

The National Kidney Foundation of Southern California (NKFSC) has worked with thousands of people who are facing kidney failure. They have also worked with their families and healthcare providers, gaining the perspective that people receiving treatment are people first and patients second. Treatment does become part of a person's life, but does not need to become a person's total life.

Knowing that adjustment to kidney failure and treatment can come with anxiety and the fear of the unknown, NKFSC first published *When Your Kidneys Fail* in 1982 and multiple editions thereafter as part of its mission in patient education. Now titled *Living Well With Kidney Disease*, this resource is designed to continue in its predecessor's footsteps, answering the need for information in order to combat the anxiety that results due to a lack of information.

This book is by its design an accessible, readily available resource. Have a particular question on a subject and need an answer fast? Turn to the Table of Contents, find your question and turn to that page for the latest information. Or, read the book from cover to cover – it is up to you. You can use this resource with confidence, knowing that from its original author through our many outstanding volunteer contributors over the years, you have their experience at your fingertips.

It is not our intent to advocate one method of treatment over another, nor does this book include all possible information about kidney failure or kidney disease. It does, however, provide enough information to help form questions that can be answered by your physician, and it contains resources to help you become your own best advocate.

Live well.

The Medical Advisory Board of the NKF of Southern California

Lilly Barba, MD
Chair, Board of Directors

Linda D. Small
Executive Director

National Kidney Foundation of Southern California

Acknowledgments

Since its first publication *When Your Kidneys Fail* has served as a valuable guide for people with chronic kidney failure. Living with this disease requires significant, often profound, adjustments in many aspects of life. Dialysis therapy alters the routine of daily life for people receiving treatment and their families. Dietary restrictions are almost always needed. Transplantation requires, in many cases, the use of potent immunosuppressant agents that increase the risk of serious infections. The personal economic impact of this disease may be enormous. A team of physicians, nurses, technicians, dietitians, and social workers is needed to help patients deal with the multiple implications of the disease.

Advances in research and in the medical and surgical management of kidney disease led to the need to review and revise this handbook. This task would not have been possible without the important contributions made by the consulting reviewers, and the kidney care professionals of Southern California.

Also, a very special thanks goes to Mickie Hall Faris, MPH, MBA, for writing the original manuscript of this handbook.

Medical Advisory Board, Education Committee, peer reviewers:

Katherine Bolden, RN, MSN
Mohamed El-Shahawy, MD
Kamyar Kalantar-Zadeh, MD
Elaine S. Kamil, MD
Mohammad Malekzadeh, MD
Scott Rasgon, MD
Judy Weintraub, MS Ed.

National Kidney Foundation of Southern California
Board of Directors:

Lilly M. Barba, MD
Laura DeLuisa
Van C. Durrer, II
Mohamed El-Shahawy, MD
George E. Fischmann, MD, FACP
Evelyn Fleishman
Barbara Gales, RN
Maggie Holloway, RN
Elaine S. Kamil, MD
Gretchen Kasai
Mahesh Krishnan, MD, MPH
Mohammad Malekzadeh, MD
Norm L. Rosenberg, CPA
Les Rosenthal
Linda D. Small
Miroslaw Smogorzewski, MD

Executive Director:
Linda D. Small

Resource Organizations

For Southern California Counties

National Kidney Foundation of Southern California
17100 Ventura Blvd. Suite 222
Encino, CA 91316-4026
818.783.8153
800.747.5527 (In California)
website: www.kidneysocal.org

Additional Resources

American Association of Kidney Patients
(AAKP), National Office
3505 E. Frontage Road Suite 315
Tampa, Florida 33607
800.749.2257
email: info@aakp.org
website: www.aakp.org

AAKP, Los Angeles Chapter
9854 National Boulevard #212
Los Angeles, CA 90034
310.364.1807
email: aakpla@yahoo.com

AAKP, Harbor-South Bay-Orange
County Chapter
P.O. Box 8
Seal Beach, CA 90740
email: mheisick@aol.com

Donate Life America
700 N. Fourth Street
Richmond, Virginia 23219
phone: 804.782.4920
website: www.donatelife.net

National Kidney Foundation
30 East 33rd Street
New York, NY 10016
800.622.9010
website: www.kidney.org

Renal Support Network
1311 N. Maryland Ave.
Glendale, CA 91207
818.543.0896
email: info@RSNhope.org
website: www.RSNhope.org

Southern California Renal Disease
Council
ESRD Network 18
6255 Sunset Boulevard, Suite 2211
Los Angeles, CA 90028
323.962.2020
800.637.4767
website: www.esrdnetwork18.org

Living Well With Kidney Disease

Table of Contents

Chapter Four – Treatment for Anemia

Chapter Five – Kidney Transplantation

Chapter Six – Diet and Medication

Diet

Medication

Chapter Seven – Adjustment and Rehabilitation

Chapter Eight – Financial Information and Other Resources

Chapter Twelve – Cardiovascular Complications

Chapter Thirteen – Renal Bone Disease

Chapter Fourteen – Advance Directives

       Ronald B. Miller, M.D., Clinical Professor of Medicine Emeritus, founding Chief of the Renal Division and founding Director of the Program in Medical Ethics, Department of Medicine, President of the UCI Emeriti Association, University of California, Irvine.

Living Well With Kidney Disease

Kidney Function

The kidneys are organs in the body whose function is necessary to maintain life. Most people are born with two kidneys, located in the middle of the back, one on each side of the spine (see Figure 1).

What are kidneys?

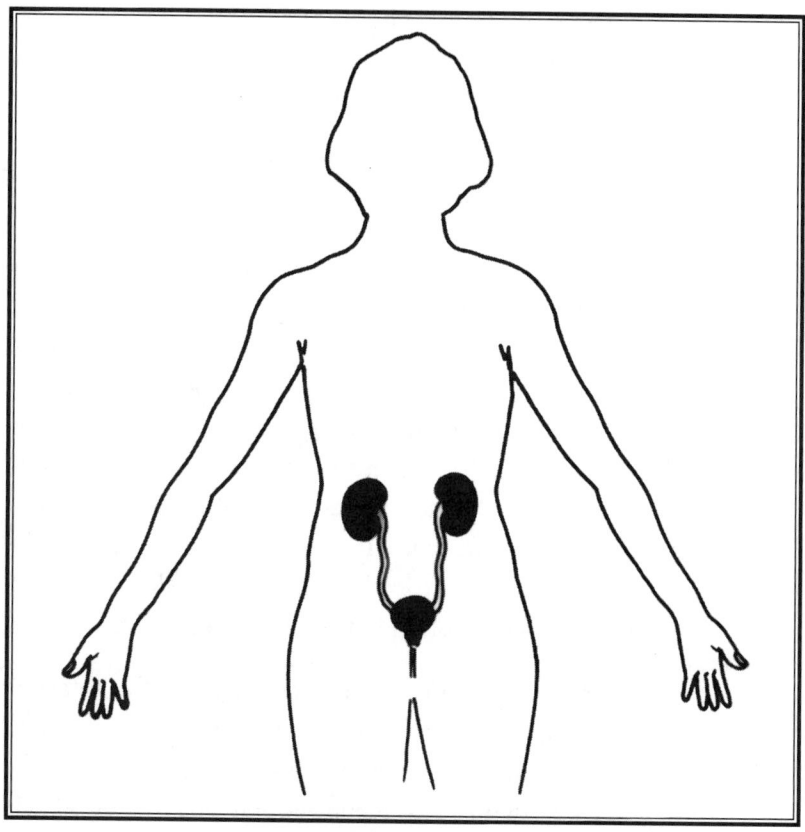

Figure 1
Location of the kidneys

What is the function of the kidneys?

Most people associate kidneys with urine formation. In making the urine, the kidneys can get rid of extra water, salt and other chemicals that the body does not need. The kidneys also keep water and other substances the body needs from being lost in the urine. The kidneys are the body's "master chemists."

The kidneys have many functions. They:
- adjust the body's fluids
- balance the body's chemicals
- remove waste products from the body
- release several *hormones*

These functions are described in greater detail in the following paragraphs.

BODY FLUIDS. The kidneys regulate the removal or retention of body fluids. If a person takes in a large amount of salt (sodium) in their diet, they become thirsty and may drink more fluid. If the kidneys are normal, they remove the extra salt and fluid in the urine. If the kidneys are not working properly, the extra salt and fluid build up in the body may cause the hands, feet and face to swell. This swelling is called *edema*. If there is too much fluid in the body, it can collect in the lungs and make breathing difficult. It can also put an extra strain on the heart.

BODY CHEMICALS. The normal kidney balances the internal chemistry of the body. The kidneys not only remove certain chemicals, but also keep other substances and chemicals that the body needs. Potassium is one of the substances the body needs for normal heart and muscle function. When one eats food with potassium in it, the kidneys work to keep a normal level of potassium in the blood. If the kidneys are not working properly and the potassium builds up in the blood, then muscle function is affected, which may cause weakness. Too much potassium in the blood can also affect the heart, at times, to a dangerous degree. Several chemical reactions in the body produce acid substances. Normally, the body maintains a healthy balance of acid. If too many acid substances build up in the body, the kidney responds by adding a *buffer* to normalize the balance. If the kidney is not working, the normal acid balance cannot be controlled, which can cause a condition called *acidosis*. Normal kidneys also balance other substances in the body that include protein. Also, certain kidney diseases result in a leak of protein into the urine, which can even contribute to *malnutrition*.

WASTE PRODUCTS. Waste products are formed from the breakdown of the protein contained in foods and from normal muscle activity. When the kidneys are not functioning, these waste products build up in the blood and may act like poison to the body. The buildup of waste products can cause one to be tired, weak and nauseated. This is sometimes called *uremia*, uremic syndrome or uremic poisoning, because urea is one of the waste products that builds up.

HORMONES. Hormones are substances released by glands and organs to stimulate a specific activity elsewhere in the body. Normal kidneys release several hormones, three of which are renin, *erythropoietin* and an activated form of Vitamin D. Renin helps to regulate blood pressure. In poorly functioning kidneys, the release of renin can become uncontrollable and can cause high blood pressure. The kidneys release erythropoietin to help the bone marrow make red blood cells. When the kidneys are not working, fewer red blood cells are made, which is a cause of anemia. Activated Vitamin D regulates calcium absorption from food and helps maintain normal bone structure. When kidney function is impaired, less calcium enters the body and bone disease can result.

How do the kidneys function? Blood enters the kidneys through arteries from the heart. The blood is then cleansed as it passes through tiny filters called *nephrons*. The waste products and fluid are filtered out, forming the urine, which is passed through the ureter and then to the bladder. When the bladder is full, the urine is passed out of the body through the urethra (see Figure 2).

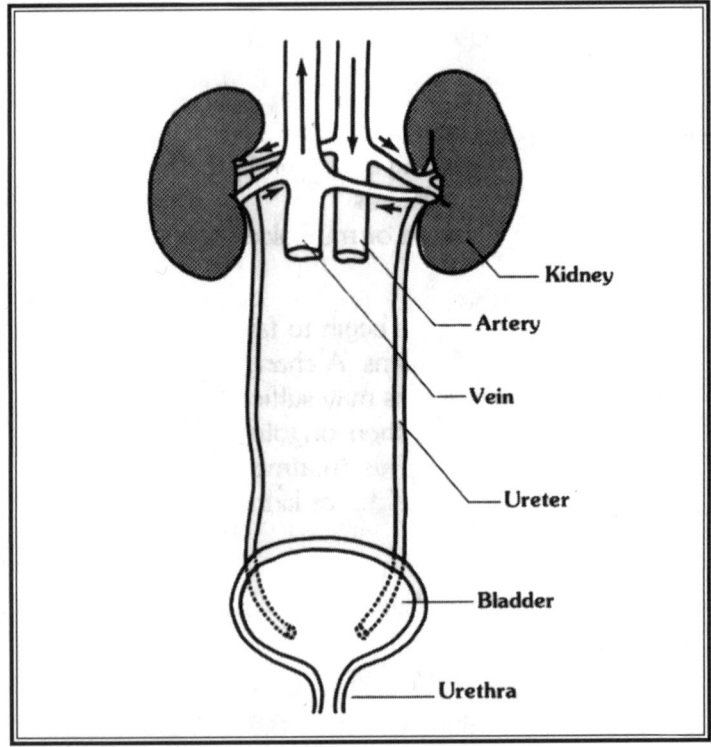

Figure 2
Kidney Function

Does everyone have two kidneys? No. Some people are born with only one kidney or have lost the function of their second kidney. If the remaining kidney is healthy and functions properly, they can continue to live normal lives. Other people are born with more than two kidneys. These extra kidneys usually do not function.

Usually, the first symptom of chronic kidney disease that may cause a person to see a physician is a general feeling of tiredness. However, many symptoms can occur when the kidneys are not working properly. Five of the major warning signs are:

What are the symptoms of chronic kidney disease?

- a change in the frequency or pattern of urination
- bloody or coffee-colored urine
- swelling of the face, feet or abdomen
- lower back pain
- high blood pressure

In young children, an inability to gain weight and height appropriate for age may be the first warning sign of kidney disease.

It is possible that a person may not have these signs even though he or she is losing kidney function. Very often physical examinations and laboratory tests are needed to detect the problem. Other symptoms of chronic kidney disease are:

- inability to concentrate
- dizziness
- inability to sleep at night
- itchiness all over the body
- decreased appetite, nausea
- an abnormal taste in the mouth
- vomiting
- weight loss
- numbness in arms and legs
- feeling of coldness
- burning sensation in the feet
- headaches
- slurred or mumbled speech

When and how should one be screened for kidney disease?

Certain kidney diseases run in families (genetic). If a family member has kidney disease, ask your physician if you need to be screened for it. Screening includes simple tests like a blood test, urine test and taking a picture (ultrasound) of your kidneys. Kidney disease is not contagious, that means it does not 'spread' by being in contact, or living with a person who has kidney disease.

What happens if both kidneys fail?

As kidneys begin to fail, initially, there may be no symptoms. At this early stage, a change in diet and the use of medications may suffice for treatment. If both kidneys fail to function, then ongoing medical treatment is needed. This treatment can be either some form of dialysis or kidney transplantation.

What is the difference between acute and chronic kidney failure?

The main differences between the two types of kidney failure, acute and chronic, are how quickly the process of kidney failure occurs, the causes of the kidney failure, and the duration of the kidney failure.

ACUTE KIDNEY FAILURE is the rapid stopping of kidney function, which can occur during a period of a few hours or days. There are many possible causes of acute kidney failure, which can include severe shock and loss of blood, possibly from an auto accident, burn injury, severe allergic reaction to certain medications, severe dehydration (especially in children), gunshot wound or extensive surgery; certain types of poisoning; certain types of a kidney disease called glomerulonephritis; and injury to or blockage of the blood vessels leading to the kidneys. During the period that the kidneys are not functioning, some form of dialysis may be necessary. Normal kidney function may return after a few weeks to several months, after which dialysis is no longer needed.

CHRONIC KIDNEY FAILURE occurs from the destruction of normal kidney tissues over a longer length of time. Very often there are no symptoms until more than half of the kidney function is lost. When very little kidney function remains, the physician recommends either some form of dialysis or kidney transplantation. The kidney function in chronic kidney failure does not return except in very rare instances.

What is the treatment for kidney failure?

As kidney function is lost, a physician may recommend drugs to control high blood pressure and a special diet low in protein and phosphorus to reduce the level of toxins in the body. They may also recommend restrictions in fluid intake and salt intake. A special weekly or twice weekly shot called Erythropoietin (EPO) may be recommended to increase the production of red blood cells to fight anemia. In young children growth hormone shots may be recommended to help children grow.

When medications alone are no longer effective and there is very little kidney function remaining, either some form of dialysis or kidney transplantation becomes necessary for survival. These should be considered months in advance of the symptoms of kidney failure so that there is time to consider which form of treatment is most suitable and least inconvenient for a person, and to prepare for dialysis or transplantation.

What are the causes of chronic kidney failure?

Chronic kidney failure has many possible causes, some of which are:
- some forms of diabetes, which can create a condition called *diabetic nephropathy*
- hypertension, or high blood pressure, which can damage the blood vessels in the kidney and reduce the blood supply to the kidney, thereby causing a condition called *nephrosclerosis*

- chronic *glomerulonephritis*, which results from an inflammation in the kidney that destroys kidney tissue
- *polycystic kidney disease*, an inherited disease, which causes the normal kidney tissue to be replaced by cysts
- *pyelonephritis*, which results from a chronic infection of the kidney
- interstitial nephritis, which is a chronic inflammation of the kidney, sometimes due to certain drugs
- systemic lupus erythematosus (SLE), a connective tissue disorder, which may affect many organs in the body
- arteriosclerosis, or hardening of the arteries
- obstruction to the normal flow of urine

There are other possible causes of kidney failure besides the ones mentioned. For more information on those, as well as more information on the ones listed, a person should talk to his or her physician.

What is End-Stage Renal Disease (ESRD)?

End-Stage Renal Disease (ESRD) has the same meaning as the term irreversible chronic kidney failure, or that stage of kidney damage requiring dialysis or transplantation.

How can the progress of chronic kidney disease to ESRD be slowed down?

It is sometimes possible to slow the progression of chronic kidney disease to ESRD. Your physician may advise you on one or more of the following:

- Keeping your blood pressure in the normal range by adhering to the prescribed diet, avoiding excessive weight gain, and taking medications regularly
- Keeping your blood sugar in the normal range
- Taking medications called ACE inhibitors or ARBs to decrease the loss of protein in the urine and reduce kidney scarring

When kidney function is reduced to approximately five to ten percent of normal, or when 95 percent function has been lost, either some form of dialysis or kidney transplantation is needed for survival. The percentage of remaining function below which treatment is required may vary with the individual depending upon the person's health and the physician's recommendation.

When is dialysis or kidney transplantation needed?

Chapter Two

Methods of Treatment

What is dialysis? Dialysis is a medical treatment that replaces some of the functions that the kidneys can no longer perform. A machine is used to cleanse the blood of waste products and remove excess fluid. Treatments must be done regularly to prevent the buildup of these waste products and fluid. There are two main types of dialysis: hemodialysis and peritoneal dialysis.

What is hemodialysis? Hemodialysis is a form of dialysis that uses an artificial kidney machine to remove waste products and fluid from the blood of patients with kidney failure. These patients must have a *dialysis access* that allows for the temporary removal of blood from the body to be cleansed. The blood is carried to the dialysis machine and pumped through a special filter called a *dialyzer (artificial kidney)*, which cleanses and removes fluid from the blood. The blood is then returned to the body. In this way, a patient's blood is continuously run through the machine and back into the body. Only about a pint is outside the body at a given time. Hemodialysis is usually done three times a week in an outpatient *dialysis facility*.

What is home hemodialysis? Some patients can perform their own dialysis at home. Home hemodialysis can be done from three to six times per week. Five or more sessions is called daily home hemodialysis. In fact, hemodialysis may be done overnight in the home or at an outpatient unit. This is called *nocturnal dialysis*. Hemodialysis is explained in greater detail in Chapter 3.

What is peritoneal dialysis? Peritoneal dialysis is another method of removing waste and excess fluid from the body. Blood is not removed from the body and pumped through a machine. Instead, the lining of the abdominal cavity (or the peritoneal cavity) is used as the filter. A tube, or catheter, is surgically placed in the abdominal wall and a specially prepared solution (called *peritoneal dialysate*) is put into in the *abdomen* through the catheter. This solution remains in the abdomen for a specified time, usually 4-6 hours, and then is drained. The drained solution (dialysate) contains the body's excess fluid and wastes. This process, called an *exchange*, is repeated several times each day by the patient. A peritoneal dialysis machine, or cycler, can be used and exchanges can be done throughout the night while the patient is sleeping. For additional information regarding peritoneal dialysis, see Chapter 3.

What is kidney transplantation?

A kidney transplant is another treatment for kidney failure. A kidney can be removed from a living relative, from a friend, or from an unrelated deceased person and surgically inserted into the patient. This is done instead of undergoing dialysis to artificially replace the patient's lost kidney function. This one new kidney would replace the functions of the patient's own failed kidneys. For more information, see Chapter 5.

When was dialysis treatment developed?

The first modern artificial kidney was successfully developed during World War II by Dr. Willem Kolff in Holland. It was initially used for short periods of time for acute kidney failure. In 1960 Dr. Belding Scribner developed a special hemodialysis access devise called a Scribner shunt, which allowed for long-term, repeated dialysis treatments to treat chronic kidney failure.

Does dialysis cure chronic kidney failure?

No. Dialysis or artificial kidney treatment does not cure chronic kidney failure, but it does allow a person to maintain life and reasonable health.

Chapter Three

Dialysis Treatments

How many people in the country receive dialysis treatment?

There are over 300,000 people being treated with various forms of dialysis in the United States today.

How long can I live while receiving dialysis treatment?

Some people in the United States have received dialysis treatments for over 20 years. No one can tell you how long you will live on dialysis. This will depend upon your overall health and other diseases that you may have.

You may not need to have dialysis treatments for the rest of your life. Many people that start dialysis can get a kidney transplant. If you get a kidney transplant, you will be able to stop dialysis for as long as the transplanted kidney works. If you have a suitable *living donor* available, you may be able to have a kidney transplant even before the need for dialysis or after having dialysis for only a short period of time. If you don't have a living donor but your health allows you to get a kidney transplant, your name can be put on a *national waiting list*. Depending on where you live, you may need to have dialysis treatment for 3-6 years before you get a kidney transplant.

What are the different forms of dialysis?

There are two major forms of treatment, hemodialysis and peritoneal dialysis. Hemodialysis is when your blood is passed through an artificial kidney and then returned back to your body. The artificial kidney does part of the work done by your own kidneys. Hemodialysis can be done either at a dialysis center or, after 4-6 weeks of training, at home.

Peritoneal dialysis is a form of dialysis in which dialysis liquid is put in your abdomen through a catheter. The catheter is placed during a minor surgery. The thin lining inside your abdomen (peritoneum) works like an artificial kidney. Peritoneal dialysis is done by patients at home, after 3-5 days of training at a dialysis center.

The decision of whether or not to dialyze at home is an individual one. You may prefer being dialyzed by trained professionals in a center, or you may enjoy the freedom of being able to dialyze at home. As with other types of treatment, there are pros and cons to home dialysis. The pros include:
- more flexibility in scheduling treatment
- time saved in travel to and from the dialysis center
- a better understanding of the treatment procedure
- more time to spend with your family and in your home
- more privacy than in the dialysis center
- if you choose peritoneal dialysis, no need for needles or blood to be taken out

The cons to home dialysis can include:
- requiring someone trained to assist you (for home hemodialysis)
- not enough space to store the necessary equipment and supplies
- having equipment in the home as a reminder of your need for treatment

Which form of dialysis is best for me?

Hemodialysis is the type of dialysis used most in the United States. However, you are equally likely to do well with either hemodialysis or peritoneal dialysis. This is especially true early in your dialysis treatments. Most patients pick a type of dialysis based upon personal preference, lifestyle and whether or not they want to take care of their dialysis. In some patients, there are medical reasons why one form of dialysis may be a better choice for them. You should work with your doctor, nurse and/or social worker to decide upon the form of dialysis that is right for you.

Do I have a choice in selecting treatment?

Yes. Most patients with kidney failure do not have any medical reasons that make one type of dialysis better than the other. So, one of the most important things to think about is how the treatment fits into your lifestyle. This is a decision that can be best made by you and your family. However, this decision should be made in close partnership with your doctor. He/she can advise you if a certain form of dialysis may not fit your medical conditions. The choice of treatment should be based upon your medical condition and input provided by you, and your family.

What is NKF-K/DOQI?

The National Kidney Foundation's Kidney Disease Outcomes Quality Initiative was created to improve patient outcomes and quality of life for people with kidney disease, including patients that are receiving dialysis treatment. For health care workers, *clinical practice guidelines* were developed to help meet *standards of care*. Many people, both professionals and kidney patients, have participated in the development of these guidelines. Guidelines have been developed in ten different areas regarding the care of patients with kidney disease. As new information becomes available, guidelines are added and updated.

It is important that you, as a patient, learn about these guidelines, as well. You are an important part of your renal care team. You can improve your health and quality of life by taking an active part in your treatment plan.

In this chapter of *Living Well With Kidney Disease*, we will include some of the key issues that you should understand. Other NKF-K/DOQI educational materials are available by calling your local National Kidney Foundation Affiliate, as well as through our National Office at (800) 622-9010 or at www.kdoqi.org.

The K/DOQI guidelines suggest it is important to start dialysis before some of the effects of kidney failure begin. Sometimes, as kidneys fail, patients become uremic and lose their appetites. This can lead to malnutrition. Dialysis may be easier if you are not malnourished before you start treatment. The decision about when to start dialysis treatments is generally based on how you feel, kidney function test results and your nutritional status.

What do the K/DOQI guidelines say about when to start dialysis treatment?

Much of your anxiety and fear is because the dialysis treatment is so new and seems very complex at first. Once you become familiar with the treatment, then adjustment can begin. You will not change simply because you are receiving dialysis treatment. How long it takes for you to adjust to dialysis depends upon several things:
- your personal and work life
- support of family and friends and
- other diseases, conditions or problems that you may have

How long will it take to become adjusted to dialysis?

After starting dialysis treatment, the amount of urine that your kidneys make will continue to decrease over time. The longer your kidneys make urine, the better it is for your overall health. There are many things that determine how long you will continue to make urine. The most important are the other diseases that you may have like diabetes, high blood pressure or heart disease. In general, patients that start peritoneal dialysis make urine longer than patients that start hemodialysis. Even if you make a normal amount of urine, you still need dialysis. The amount of waste products in your urine is low and continues to build up in the blood.

Will I continue to make urine after I start dialysis treatment?

How does hemodialysis work? Artificial kidney (hemodialysis) treatment replaces some of the most important work done by normal kidneys. First, the artificial kidney (dialyzer) helps to maintain water balance by removing extra water from the body through a process called ultrafiltration. Second, the artificial kidney removes waste products and balances potentially toxic chemicals in the blood, through a process known as *diffusion*. By combining ultrafiltration and diffusion, the artificial kidney balances the fluid and chemicals in the body and gets rid of important waste products.

The artificial kidney, or dialyzer, is made up of two compartments. The blood flows into small hollow tubes. This is called the blood compartment. Each small tube is made of a partly porous membrane (semipermeable). The second compartment is called the dialysate compartment.

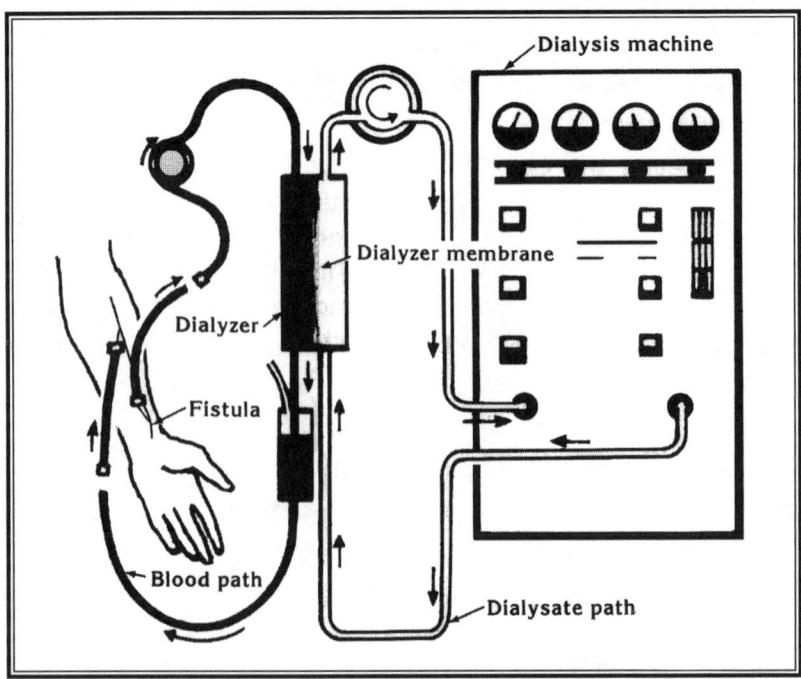

Figure 3

The hemodialysis process

A special form of liquid, the dialysate, flows through the dialysate compartment. The semipermeable membrane stops the blood from mixing with the dialysate solution and allows for ultrafiltration and diffusion. This membrane has very small holes that cannot be seen without a microscope. These holes allow some substances to move across the membrane. The holes are too small to allow blood cells like red and white blood cells, or proteins to move from the blood into the dialysate. Bacteria are too large to enter the blood from the dialysate. Figure 3 shows the hemodialysis process.

ULTRAFILTRATION is the dialysis process that removes fluids from the blood. Ultrafiltration occurs because of negative pressure exerted by a vacuum pump on the dialysate compartment that pulls fluid out the blood. Figure 5 shows an example of ultrafiltration.

DIFFUSION is the process that allows the passage of chemicals and fluids through the semipermeable membrane of the dialyzer. When two solutions of different concentrations are separated by a semipermeable membrane, very small particles or molecules in the two solutions move back and forth across the membrane. If the molecules are small and the process is allowed to continue for some time, the two solutions will become equal in concentration,. This movement of molecules back and forth through the membrane is called diffusion. Figure 4 shows an example of diffusion using solution A (salt solution) and solution B (pure water). During dialysis, the blood and the dialysate are the two solutions of different concentrations, separated by the membrane. The blood contains a high concentration of waste products. Because the dialysate does not contain any waste products, they transfer across the membrane from the blood into the dialysate.

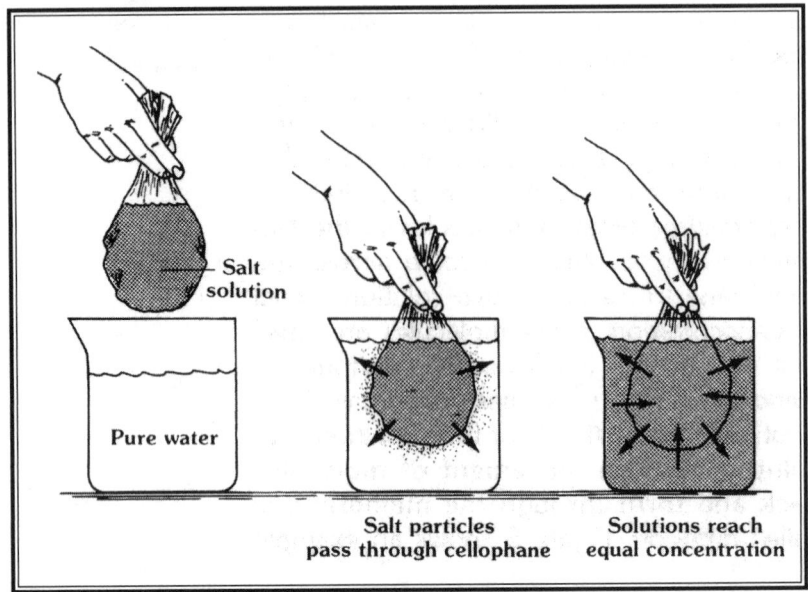

Figure 4
Diffusion

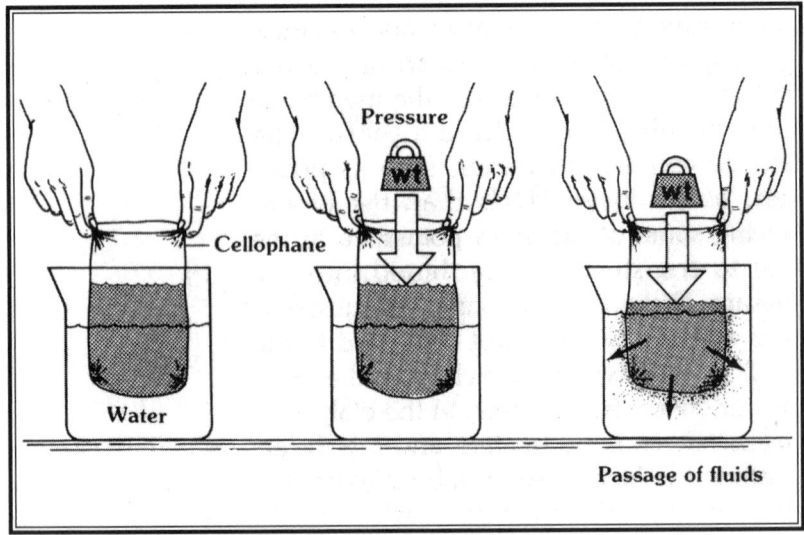

Figure 5
Ultrafiltration

Hemodialysis is a very safe procedure. Modern machines have many different kinds of "monitors." Monitors are devices that are built in the hemodialysis system that automatically and continuously monitor patient safety during treatment. If something goes wrong, these monitors will respond with a light and a noise to alert you or the staff. In most cases, the problem is not immediately dangerous to you and can be quickly corrected by the staff. The combination of the monitors and the supervision of the staff help to make dialysis treatment safe and comfortable. It may be frightening when an alarm sounds, but the monitors are designed to protect you and to make treatment as safe and comfortable as possible.

My blood has to be taken out of my body for some time to do hemodialysis. Is that safe?

Two monitors measure the pressure in the tubing that bring blood out of your body (arterial pressure monitor) and that return the blood to you (venous pressure monitor). The temperature monitor indicates an alarm if the dialysate solution is too hot or too cold. The negative pressure monitor shows the amount of suction or negative pressure used to remove extra fluid from the body. The blood leak monitor alarms if any blood leaks into the dialysate solution through a tear in the dialyzer membrane. The conductivity monitor indicates the concentration of substances in the dialysate solution. The air detector detects any air or foam that might pass through the system.

When you are treated with hemodialysis, you receive medicine called heparin. Heparin is a medicine that prevents your blood from clotting during dialysis treatment. Heparin is usually added to the blood just before the hemodialysis treatment starts. After that you may get repeated doses during the dialysis treatment. This can be given by the staff or by the use of a special pump called a heparin pump.

Why does my blood not clot when you take it out of my body for hemodialysis?

By the end of dialysis, the effect of heparin begins to wear off and blood clotting becomes normal.

Are there other medications that I will get during hemodialysis treatment? In addition to getting *heparin*, your doctor may prescribe other medications that are given as an injection. Some of these medications are *EPO*, iron and *vitamin D*. They will be given into the blood that is going back to your body.

Why do the hemodialysis machines look different? There are many different types of hemodialysis machines, manufactured by several companies. The various machines may differ in price and appearance; some are more suitable for center use than home use.

What is a dialyzer? *Dialyzer* is a technical word used for an artificial kidney. Both terms refer to that part of the hemodialysis system that contains the membrane (which filters the blood), and has blood and dialysate compartments.

Is the artificial kidney or dialyzer used more than once? Some centers clean and re-sterilize their dialyzers and use them again. Other centers use them once and then discard them. Dialyzers that are used more than once are tested to be sure they work well and then sterilized. The dialyzers are carefully marked, stored and used again only for the same patient. It must be labeled with your name and identification number and carefully checked every time it is used to make sure that you have your own dialyzer. Ask to check this before each treatment. You should ask your dialysis team if they have tested your dialyzer to see whether it still works well. You should always ask if all the sterilizing solution has been rinsed out.

How is dialysate made? *Dialysate* (the liquid that carries toxic substances away from your body) is made by adding an exact amount water to a concentrated mixture of substances. For hemodialysis, water from the city is purified extensively and then is brought to your machine through pipes. Each dialysis center routinely monitors the purity of the water being produced for hemodialysis to ensure your safety.

The concentrate contains many substances like sodium, potassium, calcium and glucose. The amount of these substances can be changed based upon your individual medical needs. If the dialysis concentrate is mixed incorrectly, you may have immediate side effects, such as vomiting and muscle aches. Most dialysis machines are equipped with monitors that alarm if the concentrate is incorrect.

How will you take blood out from my body and what is an access?

To use the artificial kidney (dialyzer), the blood must pass through it. The waste products and excess fluids are removed, and then the blood is returned to the body. There are three ways to get blood from the body to the hemodialysis machine and back to the body again. They are called vascular accesses. Types of accesses are the fistula, the graft and the catheter. The fistula and graft are under the skin (internal). Part of the catheter is under the skin and part of it can be seen outside the skin. Each access requires a minor surgery. A doctor will recommend which type of access is best.

What is a fistula?

A fistula is usually the best access for hemodialysis. It is associated with the fewest complications. A fistula is made surgically by sewing an artery to a vein. It is a surgical procedure done under local anesthesia. The fistula is completely under the skin, usually near the wrist or the elbow. Arteries are located deep under the skin and have a fast pulsating flow. Normally, veins are smaller than arteries. By sewing them together, the blood from the artery flows into the vein. The vein becomes larger and is called a "fistula." This makes the insertion of the two needles required for dialysis much easier. During dialysis, a member of the staff cleans the skin over the fistula.

The skin may be numbed with a local anesthetic. Two needles are inserted into the vessels - one to take blood from you to the dialyzer and one to return the blood from the artificial kidney to you (see Figure 6). The needles are attached to tubing that carries the blood through the dialyzer and back to the body. After the vascular surgeon creates the fistula, it often takes several weeks to months for the veins to become large enough for the needles to enter them easily. The doctor may give you instructions on how to help the veins enlarge so they can be used. Fistulas can clot or become infected. However, this does not happen often. Signs of clotting can include no vein pulsation (thrill); no sound of blood moving through the vessels (bruit); pain; and/or swelling. **If any of these happen, contact your doctor.** Signs of infection include redness, swelling and fever. You should contact your doctor if this happens.

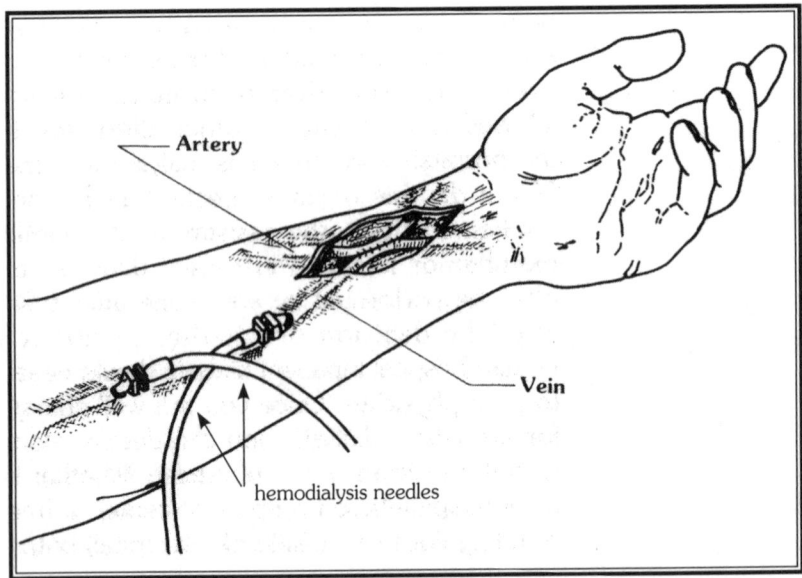

Figure 6
Internal fistula

Grafts are access devices that are similar to fistulas. **What is a graft?** Instead of connecting an artery directly to a vein, a tube of synthetic material is used to connect the two. Grafts are generally placed in patients whose veins are not able to be used for the creation of a fistula. The whole graft is placed under the skin. You can often feel a buzz over the graft if it is working well. Grafts can also clot. If that happens, you will no longer be able to feel or hear a buzz over it. Many dialysis centers do different kinds of tests every few weeks to check how a graft is working. If these tests show any problem with the graft, your doctor may send you for a procedure to fix the problem before the graft clots. The grafts can also get infected. If that happens, you will notice redness, swelling or pain over the graft, or fever. If you feel that your graft has clotted or is infected, contact your doctor.

A catheter is a hollow tube, with two channels, that is **What is a** placed by your doctor in a large vein (blood vessel). If you **catheter?** have a catheter, the tubing from the machine is connected to the two channels during every treatment. Blood is taken out of your body through one channel, run through the dialyzer and returned through the other channel.

There are two types of catheters – temporary and permanent. Temporary catheters are placed when there is a need to perform dialysis right away, and there is no other access available. Temporary catheters can be placed either in your groin or in your neck and can be used for a few days to weeks at a time.

Permanent catheters are generally placed in the neck. Part of the catheter is under the skin. The outer end comes out the upper part of your chest. These catheters can be used for several weeks until another access is ready to use. In some patients who do not have any other possibilities of placing an access, permanent catheters may be used for months or years; this access is common in children.

There are two major complications with the use of catheters. First, there is a high chance of getting an infection in your blood. It is very important to keep the skin around the catheter dry. At every dialysis treatment, the dialysis center staff will change the catheter dressing. If you get an infection, you often get a fever with chills. If this happens, you should contact your doctor or dialysis center immediately. Infections usually require treatment with antibiotics.

Second, a clot may form inside the catheter. A clot may make it difficult to get enough blood out to do the dialysis treatment. A medicine may be put into the catheter to dissolve the clot. If that does not work, the catheter may need to be changed.

The chance of complications with catheters is high; they are usually used only for brief periods of time.

What is the dose of hemodialysis? Simply stated the dose of dialysis is the amount of toxic chemicals that is being removed from your body during every hemodialysis treatment. It is sometimes also referred to as adequacy of hemodialysis. This is one of many ways to monitor how effective your dialysis treatment is.

How is the hemodialysis dose measured? Each month, your dialysis care team will do a blood test to make sure you are receiving enough treatment. These tests measure the amount of urea that is being removed from your blood, using two formulas: Kt/V (kay tee over vee) and URR, or Urea Reduction Ratio. Your dialysis team may use one or both of these tests.

Your results on these tests should be as follows:
Your **Kt/V should be 1.2 or higher**
Your **URR should be 65% or higher.**

These numbers help your dialysis team plan your treatment so that you are reaching your target dose of dialysis.

Talk with your dialysis team about what you can do to improve your dialysis adequacy. Ask them to check that:
- your access is working properly
- your dialyzer is working well
- your blood samples are taken correctly.

You also need to make sure that:
- you are there for your full treatment time
- you do not miss any treatments.

What if I am not reaching my target numbers?

Hemodialysis treatment is generally painless. If your dialysis access is a fistula or graft, you may feel slight discomfort when the needles are placed in the skin. If you have a lot of discomfort when the needles are placed, you can request a spray or cream that numbs the skin for a short period of time before needles are placed.

Does hemodialysis treatment hurt?

The way you feel depends on your health and how much uremic poison and fluid is in your system. During treatment, you may have occasional nausea, headaches, dizziness or muscle cramps. If you experience any of these, there are changes that can be made that may help. These changes include slowing down your fluid removal, increasing the amount of sodium in the dialysate, checking your blood pressure medications, adjusting your dry weight, or cooling the dialysate solution a bit.

How will I feel before, during, and after hemodialysis treatment?

You may also feel somewhat tired immediately after a treatment. One way to work on feeling well is for you to follow the prescribed fluid, diet and medications between treatments.

Are there any possible problems that can occur during hemodialysis?

Yes, as there are for almost any treatment. Dialysis is a complicated procedure that must be done carefully to assure safety. The problems during a hemodialysis procedure can include blood leaks, incorrect dialysis solution, infection and hypotension, (low blood pressure). The dialysis staff is trained to take care of these problems. They are helped by the safety features of the dialysis machines.

You can also develop problems related to the dialysis access (see pages 21–24).

How long does the treatment take?

Most people need about four hours of treatment. The length of a treatment depends on your body size; intake of fluid, protein, potassium, and other nutrients between dialysis treatments; blood flow through the access; and remaining kidney function.

How often is hemodialysis treatment needed?

Almost all patients receive hemodialysis treatments three times a week. Some patients need hemodialysis treatments more than three times per week because of their medical condition. A doctor determines how often dialysis is needed, as well as the length of each treatment.

Some new studies show that patients may do better if they receive hemodialysis treatment every day. However, this treatment schedule is new at this time and not available in most dialysis centers.

What is daily hemodialysis and nocturnal hemodialysis?

When hemodialysis treatment is done 5-6 days a week, it is generally called "daily hemodialysis". Daily hemodialysis can be done at a dialysis center (in-center daily hemodialysis). When done in a dialysis center, the hemodialysis treatment is done for 2-3 hours each day. Daily hemodialysis can also be done at home. When done at home, the hemodialysis treatment is done either 2-3 hours during the day or 6-9 hours at night. When hemodialysis is done at night, it is called nocturnal hemodialysis.

Some studies suggest that daily hemodialysis is more effective than hemodialysis done three times a week. Daily hemodialysis is better in removing salt, water and phosphorus as well as improving the anemia that occurs when your kidneys fail. However, these forms of dialysis have been done in only a small number of patients. This treatment is considered new at this time.

What can I do during hemodialysis treatment?

You can read, watch television, do paperwork, conduct business over the phone or do other activities. You could sleep, although you may prefer to stay awake to help monitor the treatment.

Do I have to go to a hospital to get hemodialysis treatment?

No, most patients don't go to a hospital to receive hemodialysis. If you require a great deal of care because of a medical complication, or if you need to be hospitalized for a medical or surgical condition, you may be admitted to the hospital. You will then receive hemodialysis treatment in the hospital.

Some dialysis centers are located inside a hospital and you may receive treatments there. However, you do not need to stay in a hospital overnight.

How are the hemodialysis treatments done? Who does them?

Hemodialysis can be done either at a dialysis center or in your own home. If the treatment is performed in the home (home hemodialysis), you and another trained person perform the procedure.

If you choose to undergo hemodialysis in a center, some patients choose to do their own treatments (self-care hemodialysis). If you have self-care dialysis at a dialysis center, you are responsible for most of your own care. A nurse and/or technician, who may oversee the care of many patients, will assist.

A nurse or a trained technician takes care of the procedure

for most of the patients who have treatment at a dialysis center (full-care hemodialysis). The nurse or dialysis technician connects you to the artificial kidney machine. This is done by either putting needles in your access or connecting the tubing to your catheter. They monitor the system while you undergo dialysis and disconnect the blood lines after the treatment is completed.

Which location is the best for hemodialysis? The selection of a dialysis location should be made in consultation with a doctor. The best location is the one that best serves your needs.

How do I find a hemodialysis center? Hemodialysis centers are located throughout the United States. These centers can be located either in a hospital or outside of a hospital. A list of dialysis centers is available from a National Kidney Foundation affiliate or you can use the internet. There are websites like www.dialysisfinder.com that may help you find a dialysis unit near your home. Your doctor is the best person to talk to about where to go for dialysis treatment.

Will I have a schedule for my hemodialysis treatment? Yes. Almost all patients on hemodialysis receive treatments on one of two schedules –every Monday, Wednesday and Friday or Tuesday, Thursday, and Saturday. The exact start time for your hemodialysis treatment will vary with each center. Most centers have two to four shifts providing treatment during the daytime hours. Some centers also have evening shifts to provide treatment for people who work.

What is a satellite center? A dialysis center in a rural area at a distance from a supervising dialysis center is usually called a satellite center.

In order to be able to dialyze at home, you should have:
- the support of a family member or significant other
- adequate room for the equipment and storage of supplies
- access to electricity and drainage and
- a good water supply

The training for home dialysis required for you (and for any person who is going to assist) involves teaching you every aspect of your care while on dialysis. In addition to being taught about diet and medications, you are taught how to prepare the dialysis machine for treatment, connect yourself to the machine, start treatment, monitor yourself during treatment, disconnect yourself, and clean or "tear down" the dialysis machine after treatment has been completed

The length of training for home dialysis varies with the training center. Most training sessions are conducted over one to two months.

In peritoneal dialysis, the lining of the inside of your abdomen (belly) is used instead of the artificial kidney. A soft plastic tube (peritoneal dialysis catheter) is surgically placed into your abdomen, often about an inch below the belly button. A few inches of this tube remain securely in place outside the body; the other end stays in the abdominal cavity. A drawing of the catheter placed in the abdomen is shown in Figure 7.

During peritoneal dialysis, sterile dialysate is put into your abdomen through the catheter. The dialysate contains very high amounts of glucose. This pulls extra fluid from your body (ultrafiltration). There is a new solution that is available, which does not contain simple glucose (but contains complex glucose, icodextrin) that your doctor may sometimes recommend. The glucose or icodextrin in the dialysis solution helps to maintain fluid balance in your body. Waste products and some other substances in the blood also move across the peritoneum membrane into your abdomen (diffusion). This helps the body to maintain chemical balance. After a certain amount of time, the dialysate is allowed to flow out of your belly through the catheter, into an empty bag. This is how peritoneal dialysis removes extra fluid and waste substances from your body. The drained fluid is then discarded. Fresh dialysate is put in and the treatment is repeated. The number of times the treatment is done depends on the type of peritoneal dialysis being used and the physician order.

Like the artificial kidney in hemodialysis, the holes in the peritoneum are very small and they do not allow

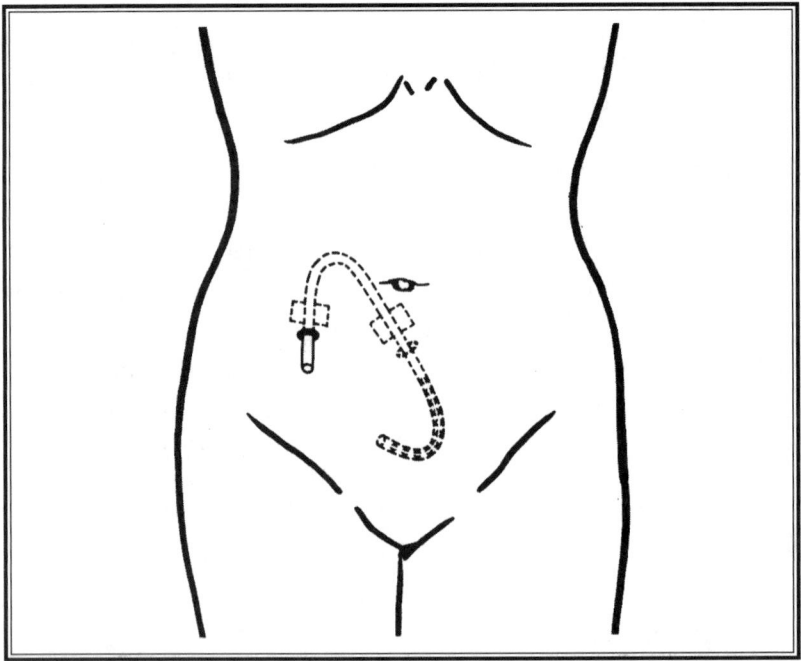

Figure 7
Peritoneal dialysis catheter

important cells like red and white blood cells, or protein to move from the blood into the dialysate. The fluid that you put in your belly is sterile. If done carefully, the risk of infection is small.

Today, two different types of peritoneal dialysis are used for treatment:

Are there different types of peritoneal dialysis?

- continuous ambulatory peritoneal dialysis (CAPD) or manual peritoneal dialysis and
- continuous cycling peritoneal dialysis (CCPD) or peritoneal dialysis with a machine.

Each type of treatment is based on the same principle, using the peritoneum to remove waste products and excess fluids. However, each treatment is slightly different, as explained further in this chapter.

Yes. Most of the time, you will have peritoneal dialysis fluid in your belly 24 hours a day, seven days a week.

Is peritoneal dialysis continuous?

Continuous ambulatory peritoneal dialysis (CAPD) is performed by you, at home, without the use of a machine. Fresh dialysate is put into your abdomen through the catheter four to five times a day, where it stays for four to six hours. This is done by attaching a flexible bag, which holds the dialysate, to the catheter using a connecting tube. The bag is then hung above the level of your abdomen and gravity pulls the solution in. The empty bag is then discarded. During this time, waste products and excess water move from the bloodstream into the dialysate cleansing the blood (see Figure 8).

What is continuous ambulatory peritoneal dialysis (manual peritoneal dialysis)?

After a certain time, a new empty bag and a fresh bag filled with dialysate are attached to the catheter. A clamp

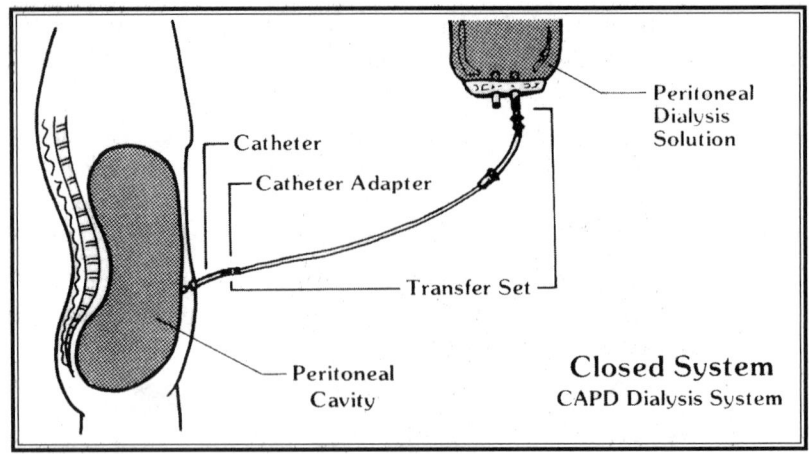

Figure labels:
- Catheter
- Catheter Adapter
- Peritoneal Dialysis Solution
- Transfer Set
- Peritoneal Cavity
- **Closed System** CAPD Dialysis System

Figure 8
CAPD process

is opened to let used fluid from your abdomen flow into the empty bag. Another clamp is then opened to let a fresh bag of fluid flow into your abdomen. The entire procedure, called an exchange, takes about 20-30 minutes. An exchange is done every four to six hours during the day. You do your last exchange of the day in the evening, before you go to bed. This exchange stays in your abdomen for eight to ten hours to allow for a full night's sleep. Most patients do four exchanges every day.

Some people may need five exchanges in a day. Your doctor may recommend a simple machine (night-time exchange device) that will do a fifth exchange in the middle of night, when you sleep.

What is continuous cycling peritoneal dialysis (CCPD) (or peritoneal dialysis using a machine)?

Continuous cycling peritoneal dialysis (CCPD) uses a machine called a cycler to do the exchanges for you at night at your home. You connect yourself to the machine in the evening or at night, at a time that is convenient to you. Most people stay connected to the machine for around nine hours. The machine does three to five or more exchanges at night for you. In the morning, the machine generally puts dialysate in your abdomen for dialysis to continue during the day time. Your doctor may recommend another exchange in the middle of the day or may let you leave this dialysate in for the whole day until you connect yourself to the machine again at night.

How big is the peritoneal dialysis machine (cycler)?

Over the last 15 years, the size of the cycler has become smaller. The cyclers are now the size of a small suitcase that can easily be put on a night stand. The cyclers come in a bag that lets you take the machine with you when you travel.

What precautions do I need to take when I do a peritoneal dialysis exchange or when I set up the cycler?

If you choose to do peritoneal dialysis, a peritoneal dialysis nurse will train you how to do an exchange and how to take care of yourself. Before you begin to do an exchange or set up the cycler, you should wash your hands well and dry them thoroughly. You need to be in a room, with all the windows and doors closed, before you begin the procedure. There should be no plants, pets or children in the room when you do your dialysis exchange. You will put a mask on and then carefully connect the tubing from the dialysis bag to the catheter. After the exchange or your cycler treatment is complete, you will disconnect the dialysis tubing and put a clean cap on the catheter.

Are there different kinds of dialysate for peritoneal dialysis?

Yes. The dialysate most widely used in United States for peritoneal dialysis contains simple glucose to pull extra fluid from your body. The glucose dialysate is available in three different strengths –if you need to remove more fluid, you will use a higher strength of glucose dialysate. The different strength dialysate bags are color coded for you to easily recognize the strength of glucose in the bag. During the training period, you will be taught when to use the various strengths of the dialysis solution.

A newer dialysis solution now available in the United States contains complex glucose (icodextrin) to pull extra fluid from the body. The rate of fluid removal for this solution is gentler and slower. It is best used if the peritoneal dialysis fluid will stay in your abdomen for 8-9 hours or longer. It should not be used for more than one exchange in a 24-hour period.

Are there any problems with the glucose in the peritoneal dialysis solution?

In most patients, there are no problems with the glucose in the dialysis solution. However, there is a possibility of weight gain (fat) caused by the high glucose, or sugar content, of the dialysate. Older people and diabetics require testing of their blood-sugar level as some of the glucose in the dialysate is absorbed into the bloodstream and can raise the blood sugar to high levels. Diabetics may add insulin directly to the dialysis solution.

Are there different sizes of dialysate bags for peritoneal dialysis?

Yes. For the manual exchanges, peritoneal dialysis fluid comes in four different sizes – 1500, 2000, 2500 and 3000 ml. The bags used for the cycler are larger and come in two different sizes – 5000 and 6000 ml. Even though the sizes of bags used in a cycler are larger, the amount of fluid that you put in your belly at a given time will be the same whether you do manual exchanges or use a cycler.

Will my belly feel distended or bloated when I put peritoneal dialysis fluid in my belly?

Most adult patients put 2000 or 2500 ml of dialysis fluid into their abdomen at a time. Some patients put in up to 3000 ml of fluid (Children will use smaller amounts). Most patients do not feel any distension or bloating with this amount of fluid. If you feel distended (bloated or full) when you put fluid into your abdomen, you can try putting a smaller amount of fluid first. As your body gets used to the fluid, you will be able to put in more fluid over time.

How will I get the dialysis bags for peritoneal dialysis?

The dialysis fluid used for peritoneal dialysis is made in factories. The dialysis center will make arrangements for the dialysis bags to be delivered to your home.

Most dialysis companies deliver supplies once a month. So, you need to have enough space in your home or garage to store the supplies. If you don't have enough space to store supplies for one month, the dialysis companies may deliver supplies every two weeks.

The peritoneal dialysis catheter is a soft, plastic tube that is placed in your abdominal cavity. This catheter is used to put fluid in and remove fluid from your belly to do peritoneal dialysis. The peritoneal dialysis catheter has three parts. The first part is placed inside your belly – this part has a coiled end with many holes at the tip and on the sides of the catheter. The second part of the catheter goes from the inner lining of your belly to the outside skin. This part generally has two anchors (or cuffs) to hold the catheter in place. The third part is outside the skin and will be the part that you see. The outside tip of the catheter is connected to a "transfer set". The tubings from the dialysis bags are connected to this transfer set to put fluid in and to drain it out.

Either a surgeon or a kidney specialist will put the peritoneal dialysis catheter in your abdominal cavity during a short, minor surgery. There are many different kinds of peritoneal dialysis catheters and your doctor will decide which catheter is best for you.

Generally, you have to wait at least two weeks from the time the catheter is placed until you can begin peritoneal dialysis treatments. However, if you need dialysis treatment earlier, you can begin peritoneal dialysis treatments immediately after the surgery. In that case, however, you will put only small amounts of dialysis fluid in your abdomen until your tissues heal.

Generally, the outer part of the catheter comes out through the skin near your belly button. However, in some cases the shape of the belly may not be suitable for the catheter to come out on your belly. In that case, an extension tubing is attached to the catheter to make it long enough for the catheter to come out through the skin on the upper part of the chest (pre-sternal catheter).

Do I have to take care of the peritoneal dialysis catheter? Yes. Right after the surgery, only the peritoneal dialysis nurse should change the bandage over the catheter. This is usually done once a week until the tissues heal. During this time, you should not change the bandage nor allow anyone else to change the bandage.

After the skin around the catheter is healed up, you will be taught how to take care of the skin around the catheter. You should wash the skin around the catheter every day with soap and water and dry it thoroughly. Many patients are taught to put a thin layer of antibiotic cream around the catheter, before putting a bandage on top of the skin around the catheter.

You should also secure the catheter to your skin. This will help prevent the catheter from being accidentally tugged on during the day or night.

Taking good care of the catheter lowers the chance of getting an infection.

Are there any problems that can occur with a peritoneal dialysis catheter? The most common problem with peritoneal dialysis is the risk of infection – either on the skin around the catheter or inside your abdomen (peritonitis). If you develop peritonitis, you will have pain in your abdomen. Usually, the fluid that comes out of your abdomen appears cloudy if you have an infection. If you have these symptoms, you must report them to the dialysis nurse immediately. In most cases, the infection can be treated at home with antibiotics. Antibiotics are normally added to the dialysis solution for peritonitis. Sometimes the pain may be severe enough to need admission to the hospital.

An infection around the catheter is called an exit site infection. The exit site will be red and/or have a discharge. An infection of the catheter's pathway under the skin is called a tunnel infection. The tunnel will be swollen and tender to touch. Exit and tunnel infections are also treated with antibiotics.

Over the last 20 years, the risk of infection has gone down. This is because of the use of special bags, the use of the cycler for peritoneal dialysis and the use of antibiotic cream on the skin around the catheter. Many patients using peritoneal dialysis never get a peritoneal dialysis related infection.

Sometimes, there are problems with the flow of fluid through the catheter. Most of the time, there is a problem with the fluid coming out. Constipation is a common cause for problems with the flow of fluid through the catheter. If you notice any problems with catheter flow, call your dialysis nurse or doctor.

How long can I have one peritoneal dialysis catheter?

For most patients, the same peritoneal dialysis catheter lasts for many years. Some patients have had one catheter longer than 10 years. No one can tell you if you will have any problems with your peritoneal dialysis catheter. On your part, you should be careful in the way you do you the peritoneal dialysis treatments and take care of the skin around the catheter. This will reduce the chances of catheter related problems.

If I do peritoneal dialysis, how much time will I be spending to do my dialysis?

You have dialysis fluid in your abdomen all the time and dialysis continues 24 hours a day, 7 days a week. The actual time spent in doing exchanges every week is about the same or less than if you receive hemodialysis.

If you are doing CAPD and do four exchanges per day, you

will spend 12-14 hours every week doing your exchanges. If you are doing peritoneal dialysis using a cycler, you will spend about 4 hours per week setting up and breaking down the dialysis system. Patients generally sleep for most of the time they are connected to the cycler.

The care of the catheter takes an additional 5-10 minutes every day.

Which type of peritoneal dialysis is best?

The type of peritoneal dialysis you choose depends on your medical condition and personal choice. Your doctor and nurses can provide assistance in making the best selection for you.

What is "dose of peritoneal dialysis"?

As in hemodialysis, getting enough dialysis treatment is very important for those patients on peritoneal dialysis. Your dialysis team will assess how much of the toxic chemicals are being removed every week. The dose of peritoneal dialysis is also measured as Kt/V. In order to measure the Kt/V, the dialysis nurse will tell you how to bring a collection of your urine over a 24-hour period and samples of the dialysis fluid that come out of your body during the same time period.

The dose of peritoneal dialysis should be measured three or four times during the course of one year. Your weekly Kt/V should be at least 1.7 if you are a peritoneal dialysis patient.

What if I am not reaching my target number?

If you are not reaching the target number for the dose of peritoneal dialysis, your doctor may recommend one of the following

- Increase the amount of fluid that you put in your belly
- If you do manual exchanges (CAPD), increase the number of exchanges. Your doctor may

recommend that you use a night-time exchange device so that this machine can do the last exchange for you while you sleep. It is also possible that the doctor may recommend that you change from manual dialysis to using a cycler.

- If you use a cycler, the doctor may ask you to do an extra exchange during the day-time.

How do I find a peritoneal dialysis center?

Like hemodialysis, peritoneal dialysis centers are located throughout the United States. These centers can be located either in a hospital or outside of a hospital. A list of dialysis centers is available from the National Kidney Foundation affiliate or you can use the internet. There are websites like www.dialysisfinder.com that may help you find a dialysis unit near your home. Your doctor is the best person to talk to about where to go for dialysis treatment.

Can I travel if I do either hemodialysis or peritoneal dialysis?

Yes. If you are receiving hemodialysis treatment, you can arrange to get hemodialysis at a dialysis center located at the place where you are traveling. If you are traveling in the United States, your dialysis center will help you find a dialysis center. Generally, your insurance will be able to pay for the dialysis treatment there as well.

If you are receiving peritoneal dialysis, you can arrange for your dialysis supplies to be delivered to the place of your travel. If the place of travel is inside the United States, your dialysis center can make arrangements for your dialysis supplies to be directly shipped there. Generally, your insurance will pay for the delivery of your supplies.

Before you make any arrangements for travel, you should contact the social worker in the dialysis unit to see what arrangements can be made and whether or not your insurance will pay for the dialysis treatment at the place of your travel.

Can I get an infection because of hemodialysis or peritoneal dialysis treatment? In most cases, infection from dialysis can be avoided by using proper sterile techniques. This includes the proper cleaning of the skin and application of an antiseptic to any point of needle entry or opening of the blood lines or at the place where the peritoneal dialysis catheter comes out through the skin.

Do I have to be concerned about hepatitis? Hepatitis is a viral infection of the liver. There are different types of hepatitis viruses; two of them (hepatitis B and C) are passed from one person to the other after coming in contact with infected blood or body fluids. The hemodialysis treatment involves taking the blood out of the body to be cleaned by the artificial kidney. As a result of this, people receiving hemodialysis treatment are at a higher risk for getting hepatitis B or C. In most cases, hepatitis causes a short-term illness that gradually clears up over a period of two or three weeks. However, in some cases, hepatitis virus persists in the body. This can lead to scarring of the liver (cirrhosis). Sometimes cirrhosis can lead to liver cancer.

In the past dialysis patients required frequent blood transfusions which increased their risk of getting hepatitis B and C. With better screening of the blood supply, the risk of getting hepatitis from a transfusion is greatly reduced. In addition, since the development of erythropoietin therapy to keep the red blood cell count up, few dialysis patients need transfusions now.

In order to make your risk for getting hepatitis B and C as low as possible, all patients starting dialysis treatment are tested to see if they are infected with these two viruses. If you are not infected and do not have any immunity against hepatitis B, you will be offered immunization against the virus. If you are infected with hepatitis B and choose to receive hemodialysis treatment, you will be dialyzed using a special machine that is only used for patients infected with hepatitis B. Your liver tests will also be routinely monitored to see if you need any treatment to help your body get rid of the hepatitis B virus.

There is no vaccine against hepatitis C. There is no need to use a special machine or be in a special area (isolation). The spread of hepatitis B and C is prevented at the dialysis center as the staff members practice universal safety precautions and isolate patients infected with hepatitis B.

What about HIV infection?

Human Immunodeficiency Virus (HIV) is an infection that can also be passed by contact with infected blood. As with the hepatitis virus, the spread of HIV infection in the dialysis unit is prevented through strict use of universal safety precautions as suggested by the Centers for Disease Control (www.cdc.gov). The staff at the dialysis centers is familiar with these precautions.

Why is fluid a problem and what is fluid overload?

Under normal circumstances, kidneys prevent salt and water from building up in the body by removing them in the urine. When your kidneys fail, salt and water may build up in your body. This is called fluid overload. This causes high blood pressure and puts a strain on your heart. It can cause swelling around your ankles. Fluid can also build up in your lungs, making it hard for you to breathe.

Maintaining fluid balance is an important goal of both hemodialysis and peritoneal dialysis treatments. During dialysis, enough fluid needs to be removed to bring the body to your dry weight, Dry weight is the weight at which blood pressure is normal, there is no swelling and all extra fluid is gone.

Patients that receive peritoneal dialysis treatment continue to make urine for a longer period of time. Therefore, you are less likely to develop fluid overload in the first few years of doing peritoneal dialysis. However fluid overload can occur whether you are treated with hemodialysis or peritoneal dialysis. You should always be careful about the amount of salt and fluid that you have every day.

If fluid overload occurs, you may need an emergency hemodialysis treatment. If you are doing peritoneal dialysis, you will need to use stronger concentrations of glucose to pull more fluid from your body.

What is hypertension? Hypertension means that the blood pressure is high. Most people with kidney failure have hypertension (high blood pressure). In some cases, the hypertension may have caused your kidneys to fail. High blood pressure puts a strain on your heart and can damage the vessels that take blood to your heart, brain, legs and other parts of the body.

Eating salt will make blood pressure higher. Removing salt and water during dialysis helps control the blood pressure. As long as your kidneys work, they will also help get rid of extra salt and fluid. This helps with blood pressure control. It is important to control the amount of salt and fluids that you take in. You also need to check your blood pressure. If your blood pressure is not controlled by dialysis treatment alone, your doctor can prescribe medications to control high blood pressure.

If you are using peritoneal dialysis, your kidneys work for a longer period of time. Your blood pressure will be better controlled during the first few years of peritoneal dialysis than in the later years. Your blood pressure is better controlled on peritoneal dialysis than if you are on hemodialysis. It is still important to control the amount of salt and fluids that you take in. You also need to check your blood pressure. If your blood pressure is not controlled by dialysis treatment alone, your doctor can prescribe medications to control high blood pressure.

Hypotension is low blood pressure. It can cause dizziness or light-headedness. During hemodialysis, hypotension may be caused by either too much or too fast fluid removal during treatment. The dialysis staff can quickly fix the problem by adding salt solution (saline) to the bloodstream. During peritoneal dialysis, if you use too strong a concentration of glucose dialysate, you may remove too much fluid. This can sometimes result in hypotension and make you feel dizzy. If you develop these symptoms, you should contact your dialysis center or staff for advice.

What does hypotension mean?

Some patients have muscle cramps during dialysis. If too much fluid is removed or if it is removed too fast, it can cause muscle cramps. The best way to avoid muscle cramps is to limit salt and fluid intake so there is less fluid to remove during dialysis.

Will I have muscle cramps?

You may have some itching. This can be a result of uremia, the level of phosphorus in the body, or allergies to medications you are taking. If the itching is related to uremia, your doctor may increase dialysis or prescribe medications. In some cases ultraviolet light treatments are given. Phosphorus is controlled through diet and medication given by the doctor. Medications may be adjusted if itching is a result of an allergic reaction to medications.

Is itching a problem?

Blood tests are usually done to monitor your condition. These tests tell about your general health. They also help check if there changes needed in your diet, medications or dialysis treatment. A group of blood tests is usually done once a month. If you are receiving hemodialysis, blood is usually taken from the dialysis tubing at the start and sometimes, at the end of the dialysis treatment. If you are receiving peritoneal dialysis, you will go to the dialysis unit for the nurse to draw your blood. These tests include

Why do I need blood tests?

creatinine, blood urea nitrogen and hematocrit. Other blood tests are performed to check the level of potassium, sodium, bicarbonate, calcium and phosphorus. See Appendix A for a table of commonly performed blood tests, including the type of test, the reason for the test and the abbreviation used.

What is creatinine? Creatinine is a chemical produced by the muscles. Normal kidneys remove creatinine from the body. When your kidneys fail, the amount of creatinine in the blood goes up. Your doctor uses the blood level of creatinine to check the level of kidney function to help decide when you should start dialysis. Hemodialysis and peritoneal dialysis remove creatinine from your body. When you are receiving dialysis, the blood level of creatinine depends on your muscle mass, amount of protein in your diet, and how effective your dialysis treatment is.

What is blood urea nitrogen (BUN)? Blood urea nitrogen (BUN) shows the amount of urea in the blood. Urea is made by the breakdown of protein. Normal kidneys remove urea from the body. As kidney function goes down, the blood level of urea (BUN) goes up. This test, like the creatinine test, helps determine how effective the dialysis treatments are.

Will I become anemic? Most people on dialysis are anemic. There are too few red blood cells in the body due to the kidney disease. This can be treated with erythropoietin (EPO). See Chapter 4 for more information.

What does hematocrit mean? Hematocrit, or HCT, is a test done to see if you are anemic. It shows how many red blood cells are in your blood. The test monitors the severity of anemia. This tests tells your doctor if there is a need to adjust the dose of medications like EPO or iron to treat your anemia.

Most patients with kidney failure do not require any blood transfusions. For almost 20 years, EPO has been widely used to treat anemia caused by kidney disease. However if you become very anemic and experience symptoms, you may require a blood transfusion, particularly if you have bleeding (as from an ulcer).

Will I need blood transfusions?

Hyperkalemia is a high level of potassium in the blood. Like sodium and fluid, potassium can also build up in the blood when the kidneys do not function well. Potassium enters the body through the diet. Hyperkalemia can be avoided by not eating foods high in potassium. There are very few symptoms with hyperkalemia. When symptoms do appear, they can be serious. The symptoms include irregular heartbeat and muscular weakness, which require immediate medical care. The best way to avoid hyperkalemia is to be aware of foods and salt substitutes that are high in potassium and avoid them.

What does hyperkalemia mean?

Phosphorus is a chemical stored mostly in our bones. A small amount of phosphorus is also in the blood. Normal kidneys get rid of extra phosphorus that come into the body with food. The kidneys keep the blood level of phosphorus in the normal range. When your kidneys fail, the blood level of phosphorus goes up. The high blood level of phosphorus can damage your bones, heart and blood vessels. Both hemodialysis and peritoneal dialysis remove some phosphorus from your body. However, it is also important that you limit the amount of foods you eat that have too much phosphorus. You may also need to take medication (phosphate binders) to prevent phosphorus in food from entering your blood.

What is phosphorus?

Your neck has four small glands called the parathyroid glands. The blood levels of parathyroid hormone go up very early during kidney failure. This occurs for many

What is parathyroid hormone?

reasons. Some of these reasons are low levels of blood calcium and high levels of phosphorus. The kidney also makes vitamin D for the rest of the body. When your kidneys fail, the body does not have enough vitamin D. The high level of parathyroid hormone can damage your bones, heart and blood vessels.

Things can be done to control the parathyroid hormone level in your blood. You should make sure that the blood level of phosphorus is kept under control. Your doctor may prescribe vitamin D injections to be given during hemodialysis treatments. If you are receiving peritoneal dialysis, your doctor may prescribe vitamin D pills. Your doctor may also prescribe a new medication that lowers parathyroid hormone (Sensipar®).

Does bone disease affect all people with kidney disease? Bone disease is a medical problem that affects most people with kidney failure. There are two major kinds of bone disease. The first type happens when the blood levels of parathyroid hormone are too high for the needs of the bone (high turnover bone disease). In the second type, little or no new bone is formed (low turnover bone disease). Both types of bone disease can cause pain in your bones. You may also fracture your bones easily if your bones are not healthy.

Are the parathyroid glands ever removed? Yes. Surgical removal is rarely done, but this is done in patients with severe disease. If you have severe parathyroid gland disease, treatment with medicines does not work to lower the parathyroid hormones in the blood. In this case, the parathyroid hormone will cause too much calcium to come into the blood. This will raise the blood level of calcium and/or phosphorus. When treatment with medications does not work, parathyroid gland tissue has to be surgically removed.

What is neuropathy? Neuropathy is nerve damage. Neuropathy can happen when your kidneys fail. The exact cause of neuropathy in kidney failure is not known. It may be related to the buildup of waste products in the blood. This build-up may cause damage to the nerves and a change in the feeling in the feet, legs or hands. Sometimes, numbness, tingling (sensory neuropathy) or muscular weakness (motor neuropathy) can occur. You may also not be able to feel the difference between hot and cold or feel pain. Neuropathy is more common or severe if you have diabetes.

Dialysis treatment can and does correct many of the physical problems that result from loss of kidney function and the onset of uremia. However, dialysis treatment does not totally replace the function of normal kidneys. You may experience long-term complications because of the loss of kidney function. Many of these complications can be treated with medication, a change in the dialysis program or possible surgery.

Are there any other medical problems that can occur?

Patients with kidney disease are more likely to develop heart disease. Some of the symptoms of heart disease can be chest pain, pain in the arm, shortness of breath, or palpitations. If you develop any of these symptoms, you should contact your doctor or dialysis center. If these symptoms continue for more than a few minutes, you should go to an Emergency Room.

Every dialysis center uses a team approach to provide your treatment. Everyone on the team has special professional and personal skills. This improves the quality of care you get. Team members include doctors, nurses, technicians, social workers and dietitians. One of the most important members of this team is you. You will have to take a lot of responsibility for your care. This includes following a diet, taking your medications regularly, and reporting unusual symptoms to your doctor/dialysis team. Dialysis treatment is a big change in your life. Every member of the team knows that this change is not easy for most

Who will be responsible for my dialysis treatment?

people. They will advise and work with you to make the changes that are necessary for your well-being.

What can I do to get the most from my treatment? Whether you do hemodialysis or peritoneal dialysis, there are many ways you can take an active role in your treatment. Remember, following these guidelines will help you feel better and live a longer and more active life.

- Keep all of your dialysis appointments. Stay for the full treatment time.
- Tell your dialysis care team if you are uncomfortable during treatment.
- Follow your special renal diet.
- Take all your medications as prescribed. This includes EPO, iron, and vitamin D.
- Don't exceed your fluid allowances and avoid too much salt.
- Ask your doctor about an exercise program.
- Learn to take good care of your dialysis access.
- Learn all you can about your treatment. Don't be afraid to ask questions.

How will a doctor take care of me? You may receive care from more than one doctor in the dialysis center. These doctors are kidney specialists or nephrologists. Your doctor will be responsible for monitoring your physical condition, checking the results of your blood tests and dialysis records and making changes in your medications or dialysis treatment if needed. He/she will also see if any other medical complications are taking place. They will supervise your overall medical treatment, health and well-being.

If you are treated with hemodialysis, your kidney doctor will usually see you two to four times every month. If you are treated with peritoneal dialysis, you will usually visit your kidney specialist once a month.

Dialysis nurses and patient-care technicians (PCTs) must have special training in order to supervise and perform the dialysis treatment. The specially trained dialysis nurse is trained to monitor the whole dialysis procedure. This includes supervising the dialysis treatments, starting and discontinuing treatments and initiating any emergency measures that may be required. The staff also includes trained technicians to assist, under the nurses' supervision, in the dialysis treatment. Other technicians set up and maintain the dialysis machines and other equipment.

What is the role of the nursing and technician staff if I receive hemodialysis?

The role of the peritoneal dialysis nurse is unique. Initially, you will spend 3-5 days being trained in all aspects of performing peritoneal dialysis. Your nurse will review your medications, perform tests to insure you receive adequate dialysis and monitor your well-being. Once your training is complete your nurse will coordinate all parts of your care, including interactions with your doctor, social worker and dietitian. You should contact the peritoneal dialysis nurse if you have problems with dialysis at home. In many cases you will be able to contact your nurse if any emergencies should occur 24 hours a day, seven days a week.

What is the role of the nurse if I do peritoneal dialysis?

The social worker is a professional member of the health care team. He/she is trained to help you and your family adjust to the possible day-to-day changes in lifestyle as a result of kidney failure, dialysis treatment and other illnesses. The social worker offers counseling services and serves as a resource and referral service. Examples of problems that may benefit from counseling services are depression, anxiety, marital and family stress and sexual concerns. Examples of problems that may require resources and referral services are:

How can the social worker help?

- inability to pay for the cost of dialysis and transplantation, hospital, doctor and pharmacy bills
- not enough money to meet day-to-day needs

- lack of transportation for travel to and from dialysis treatment
- loss of employment

Can a dietitian help me with my diet? A dietitian has professional training in dietetics and nutrition. They can help you plan your meals. This is important for patients with different diseases including kidney disease. Sometimes, dietitians are called nutritionists. The dietitian's main function is to determine any specific nutritional needs and to develop a special diet plan tailored to your needs. This may include supplements, if needed. The dietitian can also teach you and your family about the importance of diet, menus, food selection, fluid restriction and ways to adjust to your new diet plan. Many dietitians will review your monthly blood tests with you, since the tests relate to diet as well as to dialysis.

How often should my nutrition status be assessed after starting dialysis treatment? A dietitian or nurse should perform a minimal physical exam and medical history at least once every four months to monitor your nutritional status. Being well-nourished plays a large part in your overall well-being and the success of your treatment.

Treatment for Anemia

In the human body, blood serves as a liquid transport medium. It carries substances vital to sustain life to all cells in the body and at the same time carries waste materials to organs that can get rid of these waste substances.

What is anemia?

Blood is made up of fluid called plasma and of cells. There are three different kinds of cells in the blood; erythrocytes also called red blood cells (RBC), leukocytes also called white blood cells (WBC) and thrombocytes also called platelets. The RBCs are the most common cell type found in blood and contain a protein called hemoglobin that is the major carrier of oxygen. These cells are derived for the most part from bone marrow. If a person has a decreased RBC count or hemoglobin, they are said to have anemia. A doctor can detect anemia by doing a simple blood test and checking for hematocrit or hemoglobin. The hematocrit tells what percent of the blood is red cells. A normal hematocrit is between 38% to 48% but in a patient with kidney disease on dialysis, the target is 33% to 36%. A normal hemoglobin is anywhere between 12 grams per deciliter to 16 grams per deciliter. The target hemoglobin value for a patient with kidney disease on dialysis is 11 grams per deciliter to 13 grams per deciliter.

Hemoglobin in the RBC carries oxygen to all parts of the body. It also carries carbon dioxide, a waste product, from various cells in the body to the lung where carbon dioxide is breathed out. The cells in the body use oxygen as an energy source, with life ultimately dependent on it. When a person is anemic, and does not have enough RBC and consequently hemoglobin, oxygen delivery to various body parts is inadequate. This leads to poorer performance by various body organs and the patient may feel tired and out of breath.

What do RBCs do?

What are the symptoms of anemia? Symptoms of anemia include a lack of energy, tiredness, depression, and inability to exercise or concentrate normally. Shortness of breath, palpitations (abnormal awareness of one's heart beating), impotence and decreased libido, dizziness and light-headedness and constantly feeling cold are also symptoms of anemia. However it is important to keep in mind that symptoms of anemia depend on how quickly the anemia develops, with the patient feeling the symptoms much more when the anemia develops rapidly. If the anemia develops slowly, the symptoms can be minimal as the body tries to adjust. Anemia has bad side effects beyond just not feeling well. Anemia is an important cause of the increased cardiovascular morbidity and mortality (heart disease) seen in patients with kidney disease.

Why do people with kidney disease get anemia? The production of RBC by the bone marrow is dependent on stimulation by a hormone called erythropoietin. The kidneys produce almost all of the erythropoietin in the body. Once produced by the kidney, erythropoietin travels to the bone marrow where it stimulates RBC production. If a patient's kidney starts to fail, the production of erythropoietin also drops leading to less RBC production and subsequent anemia.

Does dialysis help anemia? Dialysis removes fluids and toxins from the blood stream, just like kidneys. Dialysis though cannot replace erythropoietin production. However, adequate dialysis does improve the body's response to erythropoietin. Also, some dialysis patients are not anemic, even without being given erythropoietin.

How is the anemia of renal disease diagnosed? Once a patient with renal disease is diagnosed with anemia based on appropriate blood tests, it is important for your doctor to exclude any other cause of anemia. It is important to keep in mind that anemia secondary to kidney disease is a diagnosis that is decided on after other causes such as low iron or low thyroid are ruled out.

Before recombinant erythropoietin became available in the late 1980s, patients with renal failure who were anemic were routinely treated with blood transfusions. When patients are transfused, they receive RBCs from a blood donor. In the past, renal failure patients with anemia were also treated with anabolic steroids. These agents stimulate RBC production by the bone marrow.

What methods are available to treat anemia?

Now there is a much more effective way of treating anemia resulting from renal failure. Scientists have found a way to produce erythropoietin in the laboratory using recombinant DNA technology. The erythropoietin produced this way is called recombinant human erythropoietin or EPO.

Recombinant human erythropoietin is not a drug in the classical sense. It is an exact copy of the hormone erythropoietin made by the kidneys but it is produced by recombinant DNA technology. Treatment with erythropoietin is called replacement therapy, much like the treatment of hypothyroidism by thyroid hormone.

What is recombinant human erythropoietin (EPO)?

Patients all over the world with renal failure and anemia have been treated effectively with recombinant human erythropoietin. In almost all these patients, a good response was noticed with an increase in hemoglobin and hematocrit, which means that these patients had more RBCs in their blood. This increase in number of RBCs led to increased energy levels and overall feeling better. There was a decrease in the need for transfusions.

Is recombinant human erythropoietin effective?

EPO is a relatively safe medication. The most common side effect is rise in blood pressure. Adjustment in blood pressure medication should resolve this issue. The other concern is too high and too fast an increase in hematocrit. This can lead to increased blood thickness with an increased risk in clotting. Your doctor will monitor

Is recombinant human erythropoietin therapy safe?

you closely with regular follow up of hemoglobin and hematocrit and adjust the dose of EPO if needed.

Are there alternatives to treatment with EPO for patients with anemia from renal failure?

Before the advent of EPO in the late 1980s, blood transfusion and anabolic steroids were the only effective way of treating anemia in dialysis patients.

Why is erythropoietin better than transfusion or anabolic steroids?

Both transfusions and anabolic steroids have important limitations. During blood transfusion, you receive RBCs from a blood donor. Even though stringent screening requirements have decreased the likelihood of passing on blood borne infections including HIV and hepatitis B and C, a small risk still exists. Blood transfusion can also lead to iron and fluid overload, which can have harmful effects. Blood transfusion can also lead to the development of antibodies to other people's tissue types, which can interfere with transplant in the future. Anabolic androgen steroids had limited effectiveness in treating anemia and had multiple side effects including development of masculinity and potential for liver damage.

What are the benefits of treatment with recombinant human erythropoietin?

The most immediate benefit of EPO treatment is increase in RBC count in the blood. This improves the oxygen carrying capacity of blood and increased oxygen delivery to the cells. This in turn has many benefits including increased energy, an increased sense of well-being and a better quality of life. Patients may notice increased sexual performance, increased ability to exercise, and an improvement in alertness and brain function. Anemia is also an important cardiovascular risk factor and correction of anemia has shown to improve mortality. Treatment of anemia has also reduced the need for and frequency of blood transfusion with transfusion's risk of infection, iron and fluid overload and antibody sensitization that might interfere with transplant in the future.

Your physician will determine if you are an appropriate candidate for EPO treatment – most patients are. Uncontrolled high blood pressure, allergic reaction and a rare side effect called pure red cell aplasia (PRCA) are few of the contra-indications to EPO administration.

Can all patients with anemia due to renal failure receive recombinant human erythropoietin?

At the start of treatment, the physician will monitor your blood counts closely to make sure you are responding appropriately to the treatment – not too slow or too fast. Further tests might need to be done if the response to EPO is less than expected.

Will any special tests have to be done during treatment?

Even though EPO will make you feel better, it is very important that you continue to follow the physicians' instructions regarding diet, medications and dialysis regimen very closely. If you are iron deficient, as most of the kidney failure patients are, your physician will give you an iron supplement, most likely in an intravenous form. Your physician will also monitor your blood pressure and blood tests closely.

Will I need to follow any special procedures while on treatment?

Your physician determines the starting dose of EPO that you will get based on your current hemoglobin and hematocrit. After starting EPO, the physician will monitor your response by checking hemoglobin and hematocrit at a regular basis and adjusting the dose of EPO as needed. Your physician will also monitor you for side effects including hypertension. EPO in hemodialysis patients is given three times a week intravenously with dialysis. It is injected into the dialysis circuit so that you do not have to get another needle-stick. Patients on peritoneal dialysis will get specific instructions from their physician on EPO use. Many of these patients receive EPO via a subcutaneous (under the skin) injection which is also the

What is the dose, frequency and route of recombinant human erythropoietin administration?

route most frequently used for non-dialysis kidney failure patients. There is also a longer acting version of EPO called darbepoetin alfa. It has to be given less frequently which can be an important issue in non-hemodialysis patients (patients on peritoneal dialysis or in earlier stages of renal failure).

Kidney Transplantation

A kidney transplant is a form of treatment for kidney failure. A donor kidney is obtained from either a living person or from someone who donates their organs for transplantation at the time of his or her death. The living donor can be a relative or a friend. The donor kidney is transplanted into the patient's body by a surgeon.

What is a kidney transplant?

No, kidney transplantation is a regular part of medical treatment when a person's kidneys no longer function. Thousands of kidney transplants have been performed with high success rates since the first successful kidney transplant was carried out in 1954.

Are kidney transplants experimental?

Patients suitable for kidney transplantation range from very young children to adults in their eighties. The transplant center will decide whether patients are healthy enough to be considered for transplantation.

Who can receive a kidney transplant?

It is generally true that kidney transplantation provides a superior quality of life and greater life expectancy, provided that a patient is healthy enough to be considered for the transplant surgery. The decision to have a transplant should be made by each patient in consultation with his or her nephrologist and the doctors at the transplant center. It is necessary to understand that following transplant surgery, the patient must take anti-rejection (immunosuppressant) medications for as long as the transplanted kidney functions adequately. Many people feel that life with a kidney transplant is better than life on dialysis.

Is kidney transplantation better than dialysis?

The United Network for Organ Sharing (UNOS) and the Scientific Registry of Transplant Recipients (SRTR) regularly publish success rates for every transplant center. In general, they are described as the number of patients with transplanted kidneys that continue to function, and are not rejected by the body during the first year

What do success rates mean in kidney transplantation?

following the transplant surgery. It is important to note that because of advances in the development of anti-rejection (immunosuppressant) medications, the majority of kidney transplants now survive for more than 12 years. These reports are available online at http://www.unos.org/ which can be accessed by computer or obtained for you by your dialysis center. The UNOS Transplant Living website at http://www.transplantliving.org/ is another excellent resource for patients to get information. This site provides information about what to expect before, during, and after the transplant.

Where do kidneys come from? There are two sources of kidneys for transplantation: About two thirds of donated kidneys come from people who decide to donate their organs for transplantation, at the time of their death. These are known as "deceased donors" (previously known as cadaveric donors) and these organs are transplanted into patients on the waiting list. The second source of donated kidneys comes from living donors. These may either be relatives or friends. Some transplant centers are considering using strangers or "altruistic donors" as living donors, in the same way that living donors participate in bone marrow transplantation. Kidneys from living donors have a better chance of working for a longer period of time.

Who is the "best" living donor? A kidney from an identical twin has the very best chance of success. The next best donor would be a brother or sister (sibling) that is a "full-match" to the recipient. About 25% of siblings happen to be "full matches." All donated kidneys must have a compatible blood type with the transplant patient. However, due to the latest advances in anti-rejection (immunosuppressant) medications, all living donor transplants have a very high chance of success. Matching has become less important, and this is why it is now possible for friends to act as donors.

Tissue typing is a laboratory test that determines the genetic similarity, or how good the match is between the donated kidney and the transplant patient or recipient. This test looks for protein markers on the surface of white blood cells that are inherited from one's parents. Six of these protein markers are identified and used for matching living or deceased donors with the recipient. This is also known as "HLA tissue typing." Because of the advances in anti-rejection (immunosuppressant) medications that prevent rejection, the success of kidney transplantation has improved so much that it is now possible to use donors whose tissue type does not match the recipient at all, provided the blood type is compatible. Blood type compatibility is the same as for blood transfusions. This means that in the case of a living donor, the patient (recipient) can only receive a kidney from living donor corresponding to the table below.

What is tissue typing and blood group compatibility?

Recipient Blood Type	Living Donor Blood Type
O	O, Occasionally A_2
A	O, A_1, A_2
B	O, B
AB	O, A, B, AB

However, patients on the waiting list for deceased donor kidneys are only offered organs from patients with the exact same blood type.

A high level of antibodies found in the blood means that the patient is "sensitized." This sometimes occurs in patients who received large numbers of blood transfusions or had previous transplant procedures. These patients may develop antibodies in their blood, which react with cells of the donor kidney. The higher the percentage of

What are antibodies and what does sensitivity mean?

antibodies or the more sensitized a patient is, the harder it is to find a donor kidney for that patient, because their blood will likely react with and destroy the cells of the new kidney.

What is a cross match? A cross match is a test where serum (liquid part of the blood) from the recipient is mixed with blood cells (or spleen cells) from the donor. If the donor cells are killed, this is known as a "positive cross-match," which has a negative effect on the transplant, because this indicates that the donor kidney and the recipient will not be compatible, and there will be a high risk of rejection.

What does the living donor need to do? The first step is to have the potential living donor's blood tested, to see if the blood types are compatible with the patient considering a transplant. Once it is known that the blood types are compatible and the cross match results are negative, this donor will undergo a series of blood and urine tests, and x-rays to make sure that no other health problems exist. In addition, the donor will see a physician and often a psychiatrist. If these physicians decide that all the tests are normal and the donor fully understands the risks associated with donation, then the surgery will be scheduled.

Are there any risks to the donor? All the studies of donors have shown that the risks to the living donor are minimal. There is always some risk when undergoing major surgery, but because this is a well planned procedure, it is not expected that the donor will suffer any long-term problems. The donor's remaining kidney will take over the function of the two original kidneys. The remaining kidney will enlarge in size and when tested, will be found to have virtually normal function. It is known from past experience, that people born with only one kidney, and those who lose a kidney because of an accident or a disease, live normal lives and have normal kidney function. There are really no restrictions placed on living kidney donors, although some centers recommend they avoid contact sports or other activities that could lead to injury of the remaining kidney.

If you do not have someone who can be a living donor, then you will be placed on the waiting list for a deceased donor kidney. There are over 50,000 patients on the waiting list, and it may take many years before you are offered a kidney.

What happens if I cannot find a living donor?

A deceased donor kidney is one that has been donated for transplantation by someone at the time of his or her death. After the kidney is removed from the donor, it is stored in preservation fluid and kept chilled until a recipient is identified from the list. When all the tests are completed to determine that the donor kidney and recipient are compatible, the transplant surgery is immediately scheduled.

What is a deceased donor kidney?

It is the general policy in the United States to protect the privacy of donors and recipients and not to disclose the names. Sometimes recipients choose to write to the donor family. If the donor family agrees, the letter will be forwarded to the donor family.

Will I know whose kidney I receive?

The Uniform Anatomical Gift Act made the Uniform Donor Card (or a donor sticker is used in some states), a legally binding instrument in all 50 states. This is a wallet-sized card, which indicates a person's desire to donate any or all organs and tissue, at the time of their death. Any person of sound mind, 18 years of age or older, can sign this card. Whether or not a donor card or sticker is available at the time of death, the next of kin will always make the final decision regarding the donation of kidneys or other organs and tissue. This is why it is very important that family members know everyone's wishes on this subject, should the situation ever come up. Federal regulations require hospitals to provide staff to ask family members, when a relative dies, to consider donating the family member's kidneys and other organs or tissue.

Where do deceased donors come from?

How do I get a kidney? You should speak with your physician about your interest in receiving a donated kidney. You should also find out among your relatives and friends if anyone is willing to become a living donor and give a kidney to you. You can assure your family members that a physician or transplant center will not accept a kidney from a living donor, if it is known that there are any serious risks to that donor. If a living donor is not available, then you should consider the possibility of a deceased donor and discuss this with your family and your physician.

If you are to receive a kidney from a living donor, the following will be arranged and completed prior to transplant:
- Tissue typing and cross matching of you and the potential living donor
- Complete medical evaluation of the donor
- Periodic physical examinations of you by the local nephrologist or transplant center
- Blood tests, x-rays and possibly other tests as well

If you are to receive a kidney from a deceased donor, the following will be completed before your name is placed on the waiting list:
- Tissue typing results from you
- Periodic sensitivity screening results from your blood serum sent by your dialysis facility to the tissue typing laboratory
- Periodic physical examinations, x-rays and blood tests

While on the waiting list, you must always be available by cell phone or pager, so you can be immediately notified when a donor becomes available. If you cannot be reached, the kidney will go to the next person on the waiting list.

What happens when a deceased donor kidney becomes available? You are immediately notified when a potential kidney becomes available. Once you receive this notification, you should stay close to a phone so you can receive the instructions regarding your admission to the hospital.

You will probably be told not to eat or drink anything in preparation for the surgery. You may need to be dialyzed prior to the surgery, depending on when your last dialysis occurred and the current results of your blood tests.

The transplanted kidney is placed in the pelvic area, just under the abdominal muscles, rather than in the typical location in the lower back, above the flank. (The locations of the natural kidneys and a transplanted kidney are shown in Figure 9.) The artery that carries blood to the kidney and the vein that removes blood from it, are surgically connected with two blood vessels already existing in the pelvis. The ureter, or tube, that carries

What happens in the transplant operation?

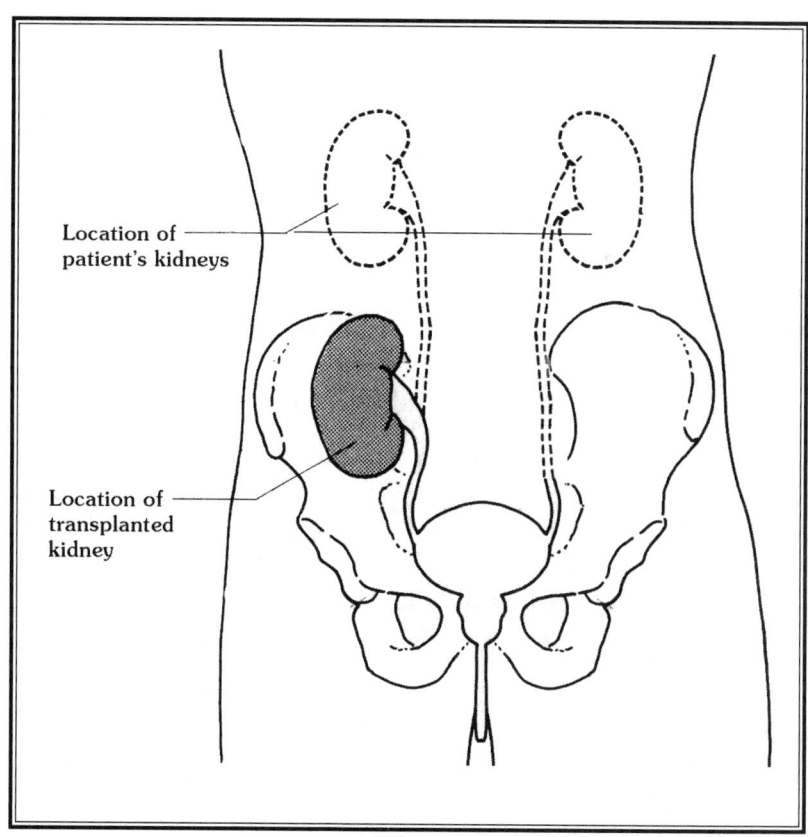

Location of patient's kidneys

Location of transplanted kidney

Figure 9
Location of kidney before and after transplant

urine from the kidney is then connected to the bladder. In surgery, as soon as the blood vessels and ureter are connected to the kidney, it immediately begins to "pink up" and begins making urine! The transplant operation takes about three hours. In very small children, the kidney may be transplanted in the abdomen, and the surgery takes longer.

Are there risks in having the transplant operation?

The surgical risk to a person with kidney failure is somewhat greater than for people without kidney disease. However, the survival rate from transplant surgery is greater that 95 percent.

What is a nephrectomy?

Nephrectomy is the surgical removal of a kidney. In a few cases, the patient's original kidneys may have to be surgically removed in a procedure called a bilateral nephrectomy, which occurs before the actual transplant can take place. The most common reasons for recommending a bilateral nephrectomy are multiple kidney infections or extremely severe hypertension.

What does rejection mean?

In the same way that the body fights bacteria and viruses that cause illness, the body interprets the presence of any foreign material, cells or tissue as an invader that must be attacked. This process is called rejection and can result in the body's resistance to accepting the donated kidney. Many people who receive a kidney transplant experience some degree of rejection. A period of rejection does not necessarily mean that kidney will stop working. There are two general types of rejection: acute and chronic.

Acute rejection is the most common form and is sometimes difficult to diagnose. In most cases, immediate treatment can reverse this rejection process. Acute rejection can be detected by laboratory tests, even before any symptoms appear. A kidney biopsy with a needle is done to confirm that rejection is present. Acute rejection may begin with fever, generalized aching, sudden weight gain, a decrease in the amount of urine produced and tenderness over the area of the transplanted kidney.

Acute rejection also can occur without any obvious symptoms. Although acute rejection is most common during the first three months following transplantation, it can occur months or even years later. Anti-rejection treatment with immunosuppressant medications must be taken indefinitely, as long as the kidney continues to function. Ongoing laboratory tests that measure kidney function are done periodically to detect a change in kidney function, which may occur without symptoms. If acute rejection occurs, treatment can include ongoing visits to a physician, and in some cases where an acute rejection is severe, hospitalization may be required.

Chronic rejection results from the continuous tendency of the body to reject the kidney. Chronic rejection does not occur in everyone, but is more likely to occur if the patient has had several episodes of acute rejection. There are usually few signs of chronic rejection, though there may be a tendency toward swelling (edema) and weight gain. Chronic rejection is usually diagnosed by repeated laboratory tests and can often be slowed with careful medical treatment to allow ongoing function of the transplanted kidney. If the patient experiences chronic rejection, he or she will need frequent physician visits and possibly some medication adjustments as well as dietary restrictions.

Yet another form of rejection is **hyperacute rejection**. This rare form of rejection can occur within minutes or hours after transplantation and can cause irreversible destruction of the transplanted kidney. Fortunately, this type of rejection is rare.

How long does it take to recover after transplant surgery? The recovery period varies with each individual and depends upon the severity of the rejection experienced, the amount of medication needed, how quickly the transplanted kidney functions, how well you tolerate the anti-rejection medication, and any complications that can occur with any surgical procedure. The recovery period could be as short as a few weeks or last a month or even longer. Many patients go home from the hospital within 5 days.

What are the chances that the transplant will be successful? Your success rate depends on whether the kidney comes from a living relative or a deceased donor. The success rate, or the percentage of kidney transplants that achieve and maintain good function, is usually better when the kidney comes from a living relative. Although individual transplant programs may have a variety of results, most programs achieve an overall success rate of 85 percent or higher.

How long does a transplant last? Many people who received transplants more than 20 years ago still have functioning kidneys, though some kidney transplants do not last that long. Some people return for a second transplant after losing their first. The length of time the transplanted kidney lasts depends on each individual situation. If the body totally rejects the transplanted kidney in the first several months, or if it fails to function, the transplanted kidney may need to be surgically removed. Then the patient returns to dialysis. Some patients choose to wait for another available kidney. Late failure of the transplanted kidney may not require its surgical removal.

Will I need to take medications after the transplant? Yes, unless you receive a kidney from an identical twin. You are required to take anti-rejection (immunosuppressant) medications as long as the transplanted kidney is functioning.

The purpose of treatment with immunosuppressant drugs is to alter the body's defense response against the transplanted kidney. Current forms of immunosuppressants medications are: prednisone, azathioprine, cyclosporine, tacrolimus, sirolimus, mycophenolate, Campath, antilymphocyte globulin and OKT3. Immunosuppressant drugs help combat the body's tendency to reject the transplanted kidney. New drugs are continually being studied.

What are immuno-suppressant drugs and why are they important?

Yes. As with many drugs, there are side effects when taking immunosuppressant medications. One side effect is an increased risk of infection, which all immunosuppressant drugs can produce. The drugs not only alter the body's immune system in its response toward the transplanted kidney, but they also affect the normal response toward invading germs, such as bacteria, viruses and fungi. A transplant patient is more susceptible to infections, which sometimes can be serious or even fatal. Signs of infection can include chills, fever, reddened areas, tenderness, swelling, cough and discharge. Any of these signs should immediately be reported to a physician.

Are there side effects to immuno-suppressant drugs?

All immunosuppressant medications can produce some other side effects. These side effects include hypertension, diabetes, increased cholesterol levels, and other specific side effects that will be discussed at the time of the pre-transplant evaluation and again after receiving the transplant.

In most cases, you may eat and drink whatever you desire. Sometimes, you may need to follow a low-sodium diet because the medications required to prevent rejection may cause fluid retention. Also, sodium restriction is required for patients with high blood pressure. You may need to be careful about calories because of a tendency to gain weight.

If I had a kidney transplant, will I need a special diet?

What are the advantages of kidney transplantation over dialysis?

The advantages of kidney transplantation over dialysis may include better health, better quality of life, no longer requiring dialysis treatments and reduced medical costs after the first year. A woman of childbearing age may be able to have children and a man may have a better chance of fathering children.

What are the disadvantages of a kidney transplant?

The disadvantages of kidney transplantation include the pain and discomfort of surgery, risk of rejection, the need for frequent physician visits and possible hospitalization due to severe rejection, the decreased ability to fight off infections which may be life threatening, some permanent conditions caused by drugs, including cataracts of the eyes, arthritis and even cancer (most commonly a treatable form of skin cancer), the cost of the anti-rejection drugs, and ongoing anxiety caused by the fear of losing the function of the transplanted kidney, and returning to dialysis.

How much does kidney transplantation cost?

The average kidney transplant without complications in the United States costs approximately $46,000. This cost covers the transplant surgeon and nephrologist's fees, hospitalization, tests, laboratory fees, medication, anesthesiologist, operating room, nursing care and costs related to organ donation for both living related and deceased donors. Individuals of any age, who receive dialysis or renal transplantation for End-Stage Renal Disease (ESRD), may be eligible for Medicare benefits. Medicare benefits cover most of the cost of kidney transplantation. Medicare also covers the cost of post transplant immunosuppressant medications. On December 8, 2003, President Bush signed Public Law 108-173, the Medicare Prescription Drug Improvement and Modernization Act. A primary provision of this act is the Voluntary Drug Benefit. Under the Voluntary Drug Coverage provision, immunosuppressant drugs are covered under ESRD for 36 months post transplant.

After 36 months, an individual may still be eligible for Medicare coverage, if they are 65 years of age or older, or qualify under disability. Some state Medicaid programs and private insurance companies will cover costs that Medicare doesn't cover. Sometimes fundraisers, charitable organizations and patient advocacy groups can assist with some of the costs that are not covered.

Chapter Six

Diet

The information in this chapter refers mainly to the needs of people on dialysis. Diet after kidney transplantation remains important, but very different from needs on dialysis.

Why must I change my diet?

Healthy kidneys control the levels of most substances in the body, including blood levels of sodium, potassium, calcium, phosphorus, fluid and protein waste products. The kidneys clear the blood of excess amounts of these substances to keep the body in balance. When the kidneys are not working well, these substances can build up to dangerous levels in the blood. This may cause you to have symptoms which include loss of appetite, nausea, vomiting, itching, cloudy thinking, and other symptoms. This condition is sometimes called "uremia" which refers to the build-up of toxic waste products. Dialysis removes some, but not all, of these waste products. For this reason, changing your diet is an important part of staying as healthy as possible with kidney disease.

Are all people with kidney disease on the same diet?

No, each person is different. The diet that a person needs depends on many things including height, weight, level of kidney function, other medical problems, and the type of dialysis they are on (hemodialysis vs. peritoneal dialysis).

What are the most common diet adjustments for people on dialysis?

The most common diet adjustments include changes to amount of protein, calories, phosphorus, potassium, sodium and fluid.

Why is protein important?

Protein supplies the body with the building blocks needed for maintenance, growth and repair of all body organs and tissues. Protein also helps the body fight off infection. Every living cell in the body requires a source of energy. The body can use protein (from foods such as meat, poultry, eggs, fish), as well as carbohydrate (breads, cereals, pasta, fruit) and fat (oil, butter, margarine) to provide energy. The body's energy needs are very important. If carbohydrates and fats are not available, the body uses protein for energy. Then, this protein becomes unavailable to perform its other functions. Also, if there aren't enough calories in the diet, the body may break down its own muscle.

Why is protein regulated in the diet?

When protein foods are digested, they produce waste products, one of which is called urea. When kidneys are not working well, urea cannot be removed from the body and can build up in the blood. A blood test called the "blood urea nitrogen" or "BUN" can determine the amount of urea present. High levels of BUN can result from excessive protein intake or from muscle breakdown. High levels are associated with nausea, vomiting and loss of appetite. Prior to starting dialysis, protein is often limited in the diet, in part to help reduce the level of BUN. Once a person starts on dialysis, protein needs are higher and protein intake should be increased. This increased need is in part due to losses of protein and/or amino acids (protein building blocks) that occur during dialysis. Too little protein can lead to malnutrition, which is associated with poor results, and even death, in people on dialysis.

Controlling protein waste products is very important. However, getting your full dialysis treatment is the best way to control waste products.

How do I know if I'm being adequately dialyzed?

One of the tests that is done each month measures how well your dialysis is cleaning your blood. This is called dialysis adequacy. The test is called Kt/V ("kay-tee over vee"). The "K" stands for "clearance", meaning how well the dialyzer cleans your blood (as well as your own kidneys if you still make urine); the "t" stands for the length of time of your dialysis treatment; the "V" stands for "Volume", a term used to describe your size - in other words, your height and weight. It is calculated differently for men and women. The Kt/V is a tool that dialysis care teams use to check if enough protein waste products are being removed to keep you as healthy as possible. Dialysis does not remove waste products the same way as a kidney transplant or kidneys that work normally. There are accepted minimum standards for Kt/V. The main factors used to figure out your Kt/V are:

- The clearance of the dialyzer used for your treatment (relates to the size of the dialyzer)
- The blood flow through your dialysis access during your treatment
- The dialysate (dialysis solution) flow rate during your treatment
- Time of your dialysis treatment
- Your height
- Your weight before and after your treatment
- Your Blood Urea Nitrogen (BUN) level (usually done before and after your treatment)
- Amount of your remaining kidney function (done by a urine collection)

Kt/V is also calculated for people on peritoneal dialysis, but the method is different.

It's important to know your Kt/V. If your Kt/V is less than recommended, your health care team will make treatment changes and offer suggestions to help improve it. The Kt/V tells if you are eating enough protein.

For more information on Kt/V and dialysis adequacy, see page 24 and Chapter Three on "Hemodialysis."

Is all protein the same? Good quality protein contains the essential building blocks (amino acids) that are needed to build, repair and maintain body tissues. Foods that contain good quality or "high biological value" protein are mainly from animal sources such as eggs, meat, poultry and fish. Foods that contain poor quality protein or "low biological value" protein are from plant sources such as breads, cereals, and vegetables. At least half of your protein should come from good quality protein. With special planning, it can be possible to be on dialysis and maintain a vegetarian diet.

Are calories important?

A calorie is a measurement of the energy value of food. A well-balanced diet provides the protein you need for growth of tissues and blood cells and enough calories to meet the body's energy needs. When enough calories are present in the diet, the body does not rely on protein as an energy source. Protein is then able to perform other important functions, such as growth and healing. When you eat more calories than you need, the body stores extra calories as fat. Stored fat can be used for energy when you eat fewer calories than you need. Calorie requirements depend on age, height, weight, activity level and your other medical problems. If you are on peritoneal dialysis, some calories will be absorbed from your dialysate solution. The amount absorbed can vary considerably, depending on the strength of the solution (sugar content of the solution) that you use. This extra sugar can result in weight gain. This weight gain can be controlled with exercise and changes in your diet. A dietitian will work with you to plan a diet that meets your needs.

What is potassium and why is it important?

Potassium is a mineral needed for normal function of nerves and muscles. Since the heart is a muscle, the amount of potassium in the blood affects the beating of the heart. When kidney function is normal, extra potassium comes out in the urine. When the kidneys are not functioning properly, potassium can build up in cells and in the blood. Although dialysis removes potassium, it does not work as well as normal kidneys. Therefore, blood potassium can become too high. High levels can cause abnormal heartbeats and can even cause the heart to stop beating. In addition, certain medications and some medical conditions may cause potassium levels to go up. You may need to limit high potassium foods in your diet. Potassium control may be more important in people on hemodialysis, compared to people on peritoneal dialysis. However, every person is different. A dietitian will give you information about potassium in foods and work with you on your potassium needs.

Which foods contain a lot of potassium?

Some foods high in potassium are potatoes, dark green leafy vegetables, most citrus fruits, bananas, avocados, nuts, dried beans and peas. Salt substitutes, which contain potassium chloride, are also very high in potassium.

Can potassium be removed from food?

Yes. Some of the potassium from certain foods, such as potatoes, sweet potatoes, carrots, beets, and rutabagas, can be removed. This is done by peeling and slicing the foods into small pieces (1/8 inch) and then soaking them in large amounts of water. For more detailed instructions, check under patient information on potassium at www. kidney.org.

What happens if I eat too much or too little potassium?

Usually, there are no obvious warning signs when the blood potassium is high. High potassium levels or hyperkalemia can be very serious and cause the heart to stop beating.

What else can affect potassium levels?

Following a proper diet will help control your potassium. Your doctor will check your potassium level regularly. Certain medications can add to high potassium. People on dialysis get rid of large amounts of potassium through bowel movements. Constipation, in people with kidney disease, can cause high potassium. Let your doctor know if constipation is a problem.

Low potassium levels or hypokalemia can sometimes make you feel weak and can cause irregular heartbeats. Low potassium levels can be corrected with proper diet, or your physician may prescribe potassium supplements if necessary.

What is sodium?

Sodium is an important mineral found in almost all foods. It is found in the body's tissues and helps to regulate body fluid and blood pressure.

Are sodium and salt the same thing?

Not exactly. Salt does contain sodium, but it also contains chloride. About 40% of table salt is sodium. All foods contain some sodium, even if they do not have added salt.

Is sodium control a part of the diet?

Yes, for most people. If you have high blood pressure (hypertension) or excessive fluid in the body (edema), it is important to restrict sodium intake. In most cases, when the kidneys are not functioning, sodium cannot be excreted or eliminated normally. The excess sodium can cause thirst and build-up of excess fluid in the body. This can cause extra strain on your heart and may cause high blood pressure.

What foods contain a lot of sodium?

The most common source of sodium in the diet is table salt. Foods high in sodium include cured, processed and smoked meats, such as ham, bacon, sausage and cold cuts; foods that are salty to the taste, such as potato chips, pretzels, corn chips, salted nuts and pickles, certain condiments such as prepared mustard, catsup, monosodium glutamate, steak sauces, soy sauce and most canned and packaged soups and entrees. Becoming familiar with the sodium content of foods is helpful. Be sure to read the food labels on packages.

What happens if I eat too much sodium?

If you eat extra sodium you may develop:

- Sudden weight gain
- Puffiness or swelling of your face, feet, legs or abdomen (edema)
- Difficulty in breathing because of extra fluid in the blood vessels and lungs
- A feeling of being bloated

Excess sodium can also cause high blood pressure, which is not always obvious. Although dialysis removes sodium and fluid, there are limits as to how much can safely be removed during a hemodialysis treatment. If there is too much fluid to remove at one time, muscle cramping and sudden drops in blood pressure can occur and make the dialysis session much more difficult and uncomfortable. With peritoneal dialysis, there is usually more flexibility with sodium and fluid intake, since the dialysis can be more easily adjusted to remove varying amounts of sodium and fluid.

Is it important to control fluid intake?

Yes. Properly functioning kidneys prevent fluid in your body from building up by removing the excess fluid as urine. When your kidneys are not functioning, fluid can accumulate in your tissues and bloodstream and may place a strain on your heart as well as cause high blood pressure. It can also collect in your lungs making it difficult to breathe.

I still make a normal amount of urine. Will that change?

Yes, that's possible. Kidney function can continue to decline, even after you've started dialysis. Over time, the amount of urine you make will probably go down as well. Some people on dialysis eventually make no urine.

The amount of fluid is different for every person. It depends largely on how much urine your kidneys are making and what type of dialysis you are using. Your physician or dietitian will advise you on how much fluid is right for you. Even though many foods contain fluid, most people count any fluid that is liquid at room temperature as part of their daily fluid intake. This would include popsicles, Jell-O™, and soups as well as water and other beverages. Weighing yourself each day is a good way to help check your fluid intake. Gaining less than 2 kilograms (about 4 pounds) is a reasonable weight gain for most adults in a 2-day period between hemodialysis treatments.

How much fluid can I have each day?

The term "dry weight" is often used by physicians and other staff. Dry weight is defined as the weight below which blood pressure drops too low – or what someone weighs once all excess fluid has been removed by a dialysis treatment. Dry weight may need to be adjusted from time to time as a person gains or loses actual body weight (muscle or fat).

What does "dry weight" mean?

The element found most in the body is calcium. Most of the body's calcium is in bones and teeth, but it is an important part of blood as well. Phosphorus is the second most common element and is found in bone as well as in every cell in the body. The body cannot use calcium without a usable form of Vitamin D. One of the things healthy kidneys do is help change the Vitamin D from food and sunlight to a usable or "active" form. In kidney disease, Vitamin D levels decrease and at the same time phosphorus is retained. This happens because the kidney is less able to get rid of excess phosphorus. This combination of low Vitamin D and excess phosphorus causes a drop in blood calcium levels. In an effort to return

Why are calcium and phosphorus important for people on dialysis?

blood calcium levels back to normal, the body calls upon a gland located in your neck area called the parathyroid gland.

I've never heard of the parathyroid gland. What does it do?

The main job of the parathyroid gland is to regulate the amount of calcium in the body. If the parathyroid gland senses that the blood calcium is low (as can happen with kidney disease) it starts to make and release a hormone called parathyroid hormone or "PTH". The PTH goes to three organs in the body in an effort raise blood calcium level.

1. It tells the bones to release calcium.
2. It tells the intestine to absorb more calcium from the diet.
3. It tells the kidneys to hold on to calcium (instead of letting it pass into the urine). It also tells the kidney to help make more active Vitamin D.

But in kidney disease this system can go "haywire". Too much PTH can be made and released. High levels of PTH can cause a certain type of bone disease, which can be very painful and cause problems with daily activities. It can also cause blood calcium levels (and phosphorus levels) to get too high. It can even cause serious problems with the heart and blood vessels and is associated with increased risk of cardiovascular disease and death in people on dialysis.

What can I do about it?

Fortunately there are medications that can control and help prevent these complications. But the main things you can do are to control your phosphorus and calcium levels with diet and medication.

Foods high in phosphorus include milk and other dairy products, beans, nuts, and seeds. Just about all foods contain some phosphorus, so it's impossible to avoid it completely.

What foods are high in phosphorus?

Yes, your physician will probably prescribe a medication called a "phosphate binder." Phosphate binders are to be taken with meals and snacks. They bind the phosphorus in your foods so you get rid of it in your stools, and blood levels remain normal.

Is there anything else I can do to control my phosphorus?

Certain vitamins are removed by dialysis. Other vitamins may work a bit differently in people on dialysis. Others should be avoided or limited. For these reasons, a special type of multivitamin will be prescribed by your physician that will meet your special needs. In addition, your physician may prescribe an "active" form of Vitamin D, which is given during the hemodialysis treatment or by mouth in people on peritoneal dialysis.

What about vitamins?

Alcoholic beverages can be included in the diet for people with kidney disease. However, certain medications can interact with alcohol, so it's important to check with your physician first.

Can I drink alcohol?

It is possible to combine a diabetic diet with your new diet. Insulin is normally processed by the kidney. In kidney disease, whatever insulin you inject or your body may be making tends to stay in your body much longer. So for many people with diabetes, blood sugar may be a bit easier to control. If you are on peritoneal dialysis, your healthcare team will help you manage the extra sugar that will be coming from your dialysate solution.

I am diabetic. How can I follow that diet and my new one for dialysis?

What happens to my diet after I receive a transplant? With a kidney transplant, diet is an important part of your health and well being. Long-term issues for most people with a transplant include cholesterol and blood pressure control, and avoidance of excess weight gain by diet and exercise. Adequate calcium, vitamin D, and phosphorus are important to maintain healthy bones and help prevent osteoporosis.

Other issues, related to your needs will be reviewed with you by a dietitian when you receive your transplant.

I have been told I am "anemic." Should I eat foods high in iron? Anemia is a term that usually refers to not having enough red blood cells. Healthy kidneys normally make a hormone called erythropoietin, which causes your bone marrow to make red blood cells. In people on dialysis, anemia can be due to too little of this hormone. Erythropoietin can be given by injection or during dialysis. People on dialysis can also be iron deficient. Your physician will check your iron stores regularly. Your doctor may order intravenous iron during your dialysis treatment or oral iron. The iron from foods tends to be poorly absorbed. As long as you are able to take intravenous or oral iron, there is no reason to try to increase high iron foods in your diet. In addition, adequate nutrients, such as vitamin B12 and folic acid will help you build red blood cells. (See "Anemia" Chapter.)

Where can I go to find help in planning my menu? The dietitian at your dialysis unit can be a very useful resource in figuring out what to eat. In addition there are numerous websites and cookbooks that have helpful information on diet for people with chronic kidney disease. (See appendix C.)

Yes, definitely. With a little careful planning you can still go to your favorite restaurants. Choose entrees without sauces, which may be high in sodium. Low potassium vegetables and fruits are also a good choice. A piece of French or Italian bread would round out a healthy restaurant meal for most people on dialysis.

Can I still eat out in restaurants?

If you have high cholesterol, limiting foods that are high in saturated fats (mainly animal fats as found in meat, cheese) may help lower the "bad" or LDL cholesterol. Also avoiding foods that contain "trans-fats" (found in vegetable shortening, some margarines, crackers, candies, baked goods, cookies, snack foods, fried foods, salad dressings, and many processed foods) can help lower LDL. Good types of fats are found in olive oil and canola oil, foods that contain plant sterols can also help control cholesterol. If you are overweight, achieving your "ideal" body weight can have a positive affect on cholesterol. Exercise can also help lower the bad cholesterol and raise the "good" or HDL, cholesterol. A dietitian can help you combine a cholesterol-lowering diet with the medications necessary because of your kidney disease.

My doctor has told me my cholesterol is high. How can I help lower my cholesterol and follow my diet?

Yes. Exercise is an important part of the overall health and well being in all people, including people on dialysis. Exercise can help control blood pressure and cholesterol, maintain bones, and control blood sugar in people with diabetes. It's good for your heart and for your entire body, and can help you maintain a positive attitude. Your physician can help give you guidelines as to what type and how much exercise is right for you.

Can people on dialysis exercise?

Medication

What medications will I need? In addition to a special diet, the doctor will prescribe medications. The medications are taken for a variety or reasons. This may include lowering your blood pressure, controlling issues caused by kidney disease such as parathyroid and calcium problems, preventing too much phosphate in your blood and increasing the amount of red blood cells. A list of some of the most common types of medication, their brand names and their purpose has been included in Appendix E. This list includes only some of the most common medications used to deal with conditions related to kidney disease. Your doctor may prescribe other drugs not listed. You should know about all the medications you are using. You should know about the good effect the medication may have on your health as well as about the possible side effects.

What are phosphate binders? Phosphate (phosphorus) binders are used to prevent phosphorus from going into the blood. This happens by binding phosphorus in the intestines. Phosphorus is present in most foods. Therefore, the binders are usually ordered to be taken just before or while eating a meal or snack. Once the phosphorus is bound it passes out of the body in the stool. The doctor will ask you not to take any other medications at the same time you take the phosphate binders. Taking other medications with the phosphate binders may prevent the other medications from being absorbed into your body. In general, phosphate binders contain either calcium or other elements such as aluminum, lanthanum or resins. Other new phosphate binders may be developed in the future. The type of phosphate binder you take is important and must be taken with the doctor's approval.

What are calcium supplements? Calcium tablets increase the amount of calcium in the blood and body. They also act as antacids and phosphate binders. The tablets are taken by mouth. You usually should not take more than 2 grams (2000 mg) of elemental calcium per day if you have severe kidney disease or are on dialysis. Look for the words "elemental calcium" on your calcium supplement label.

Vitamin D and its active metabolites (like calcitriol) cause the body to absorb calcium from food and place it in the bones. It also controls the production of parathyroid hormone. Since the kidney is the major source of active Vitamin D metabolites, patients with decreased kidney function may need extra calcitriol. Vitamin D and calcitriol come in capsules which are taken by mouth. Other active Vitamin D metabolites can be also given into a vein or through the hemodialysis tubing. Depending on your blood calcium level, parathyroid hormone level, and Vitamin D level, your doctor may or may not order this medication for you.

What is vitamin D and what does it do?

Controlling your blood pressure is very important. A good blood pressure can decrease complications such as stroke, further kidney damage and heart attack. This is true in the general population as well as in those with kidney disease. A doctor may prescribe blood pressure medications to lower your blood pressure. Another type of medication may be ordered to make your heart beat stronger, slower, and more regular.

Will I need any medications for my heart or blood pressure?

Control of lipids such as cholesterol and triglycerides is also helpful in decreasing cardiovascular complications. The most common lipid lowering medications are called statins. Statins decrease cholesterol production in the liver. Other medications may lower the amount of lipids absorbed from your diet. Statins are prescribed under close physician supervision. Occasionally statins may case liver or muscle problems.

Can I use Viagra®? Sexual dysfunction is a common problem in people with kidney disease, especially people on dialysis. There are many reasons why this can happen. Your doctor will need to examine you and discuss health and social factors. Some medications may also cause sexual dysfunction. Viagra® or other medications can be used to treat impotence in people with kidney failure. The medication is given after careful evaluation by a doctor.

What drugs promote red blood cell production? Anemia in people with kidney diseases is usually caused by a lack of the hormone, erythropoietin (EPO). EPO is produced by the kidney. EPO supports the making of red blood cells. Recombinant human EPO is now available and is used for most people on dialysis. If needed, EPO can be used for people with other stages of kidney failure. It can be given directly into the vein (usually through the dialysis tubing) or injected under the skin.

Folic acid is necessary for normal red blood cell production. Folic acid is removed from the blood during hemodialysis treatment. Therefore, folic acid must be replaced to avoid anemia. You may be asked to take a folic acid tablet every day.

You may also need iron medications for a normal blood iron level. An adequate amount of iron is needed for normal red blood cell production.

You may need to be taking all of these medications to make enough red blood cells and correct anemia. The use of these medications in people with kidney failure have made the need for blood transfusions uncommon.

What do analgesics do? Analgesics are medications that relieve pain. Some analgesics also reduce fever. Tylenol™ is an example of an analgesic. Nonsteroidal anti-inflammatory drugs (NSAID) such as ibuprofen (Motrin®, Advil®) are another kind of analgesic. NSAID's may worsen kidney function in already damaged kidneys. In addition, NSAID's and aspirin may cause bleeding and should not be taken without the advice of your kidney doctor.

Will I need antibiotics?

An antibiotic is a medication that either stops the growth of bacteria or kills bacteria. You may, on occasion, have an infection that requires antibiotics. Antibiotics can be given as a pill or as an injection. The type of antibiotic you get will depend on the kind of infection you have. The dose of some antibiotics may need to be changed in patients with kidney disease. Some broad-spectrum antibiotics may cause damage to "good" intestinal bacteria and cause diarrhea. If you have diarrhea while you are taking an antibiotic, call your doctor to get immediate attention and treatment.

Will I need laxatives?

Some of your medications may cause constipation. Stool softeners, dietary fiber or fiber medication act to soften the stool. Some laxatives cause the bowel to be more active. The doctor may recommend that you take a stool softener or order a laxative as some of your other medication may cause constipation.

Will I need vitamin supplements?

Most people with kidney failure require vitamin supplements. Supplements are used to replace any vitamins removed during dialysis or add vitamins that are not in your diet. There are many brands of vitamins, but most contain folic acid, Vitamin C and the Vitamin B complex. These supplements are the most dialyzable. Vitamin supplements should be taken under the supervision of your kidney doctor. Multivitamins containing large amounts of vitamin A, E or C should be avoided. Your doctor may order a special vitamin made especially for people with kidney disease.

Chapter Seven

Adjustment and Rehabilitation

How will having kidney failure change my life? This question is difficult to answer because each person reacts differently to their kidney failure and treatment. Learning to live with dialysis may be a minor adjustment or may demand a major change to lifestyle or even philosophy. Any important change in your life requires altering habits, priorities, schedules and outlook. Each person receiving treatment for kidney failure is an individual and that individuality remains after kidney function is lost.

Should I expect some emotional problems as a result of kidney failure? Most people with chronic illness experience some degree of depression and anxiety. Since kidney failure and treatment is a chronic condition, *not* a terminal one, you may also experience feelings of sorrow, grief, confusion, fear and even anger. These feelings are normal and many people going through what you are will also have these feelings. As you become familiar and comfortable with treatment, your ability to deal with these feelings and concerns will increase, and kidney failure and treatment will become a part of your lifestyle.

Is depression normal? Most people experience depression at some point in their lives. Depression, or feelings of sadness, unhappiness and despair, can occur with stress, loss and illness. Depression can cause a loss of appetite, decreased interest in sex and difficulty in sleeping. One way to deal with depression is to talk about it; usually, talking about it helps people to understand why they are depressed. It may help to communicate with family and friends and to speak with the dialysis unit social worker about these feelings. In many cases, understanding the depression helps to deal with the problem causing it.

What is anxiety? Anxiety is uneasiness or apprehension concerning an anticipated event or problem. If a person is anxious, they may have excessive perspiration, rapid pulse and heart rate, tiredness, irritability or agitation. Very often, the cause of anxiety cannot be determined. Many people who have a chronic illness experience some degree of anxiety. Like depression, the best way to deal with anxiety is to talk it through with someone – a friend, a family member, a minister, the social worker or other mental health professional.

There is no single way of coping with kidney failure and treatment. There are, however, several suggestions that other people with kidney failure have made to ease adjustment to chronic illness and treatment, including education about kidney failure and treatment, physical fitness, communication in maintaining important personal relationships and motivation to complete projects and goals.

How do I cope?

Education or information about kidney failure and selected treatment is very important. Knowledge of what is happening inside your body, the reaction to dialysis, why medication is needed and why certain foods and fluids must be restricted is crucial to your overall understanding of what is happening. The feeling of helplessness and dependency on the medical staff can be reduced by knowing and understanding kidney failure and treatment. Putting this knowledge to use will help you to feel better and can give you a sense of being in control of your own life. Fears and anxieties can be the result of lack of information. The unknown, which we all fear, can become known through education. Speaking with others, reading current literature and searching the internet can all be excellent sources of information and education regarding kidney failure and treatment. The Life Options Rehabilitation Program has an educational component called "Kidney School" that can be accessed through the internet at www.kidneyschool.org.

Physical fitness should be important to everyone with or without kidney disease. Mild and regular exercise can help rebuild strength, help insomnia and anemia and strengthen bones and muscles. A physical fitness and exercise program developed with the help of a physician can give you a feeling of accomplishment and overall well-being.

Communication is one way to maintain important personal relationships. Talking things through with your partner, family members and friends is very important in maintaining relationships. Sharing feelings, including that of fear and anger, and other concerns, with others not only helps you feel better, it will also help your family and friends to understand and accept what you are experiencing. Closing out those people important to you can hurt the relationship by making them feel no longer needed or wanted. Ongoing communication, like education, may help you to become aware of your feelings. Once you are aware of your own feelings, you can begin to accept kidney disease as an unfortunate, but challenging, part of life and you can continue to enjoy life.

Motivation, setting personal goals, completing projects and continuing to lead life as close as possible to the way you did before kidney failure is very important. Continuing enjoyable activities, being with loved ones and continuing to plan your life should not change with kidney disease. Most people's feelings of self-esteem or self-worth depend on what they do and accomplish. Although kidney disease and treatment can change some external aspects of your life, your essential worth and value to yourself and others can and should remain unchanged.

Your emotional state can affect your physical health and, in the case of kidney disease, can affect medical treatment and progress. If your emotional state or mental attitude is positive, you will most likely do well on dialysis. If, however, you are having a difficult time adjusting, or had problems prior to the kidney failure, you may not do as well on dialysis as someone with a positive mental outlook.

Will my mental attitude affect my physical health?

Family members face many of the emotional stresses and problems that you do, including depression, anxiety, concern for life expectancy, concern about finances, difficulty in expressing honest feelings and concern over sexual competence. In some cases, discussion groups, in which family members express their concerns and provide mutual emotional support, can help your family to adapt to your illness. The social worker can provide more information.

Will my illness affect my marriage and family?

In some cases, uremia, the building up of waste products in the bloodstream between dialysis treatments, can affect thinking. Sometimes, a person may experience difficulty in remembering things, inability to concentrate and confusion. On rare occasions, they may lose contact with reality or experience hallucinations. Seeing, hearing, tasting, feeling or smelling things that do not exist can be very frightening. If this happens, it is important for you to tell your physician. Some people who experience hallucinations do not tell anyone for fear that they are losing their minds, when in reality, the hallucinations can be caused by inadequate dialysis treatments, the need for medications or by fever and infection (delirium).

Can kidney disease affect my thinking?

Sometimes your desire for sexual activity, or sexual appetite, changes with chronic illness. The ability to enjoy sex, on the part of the male or female, depends on you as an individual. Impotence, or the inability of a male to have an erection or to maintain an erection, can occur.

Can I still enjoy sex?

Problems with ejaculation are also a possibility. However, your ability to participate in sexual activity and to enjoy sex is still possible. If you find your sex life changing, talk to your physician or social worker, because these problems may be treatable. Very often, the stress and anxiety related to kidney failure and treatment can affect your sexual appetite and ability to enjoy sex. Taking good care of yourself, including following your dialysis prescription, not smoking, exercising and remaining active can contribute to a more satisfying sex life.

Can I still get pregnant while receiving dialysis treatment or after a kidney transplant?

Yes. Although many women on dialysis have their menstrual cycle disrupted by kidney failure, there are women who have had pregnancies. Women on dialysis are usually advised to prevent pregnancy because of the high risk of potential complications. Pregnant women who are on dialysis may experience high blood pressure and other complications that may result in miscarriage, premature delivery, stillbirths, and other risks to the developing fetus. Pregnant women who are on dialysis are often dialyzed daily and must be carefully monitored. It is recommended that women who want to have children use contraception while requiring dialysis and plan to become pregnant at least one year or more after transplant. When you plan a pregnancy after transplantation, work with your transplant physician to adjust your transplant medications to ones that are more compatible with a pregnancy.

Can I father a child while receiving dialysis treatment or after transplant?

Yes. There are men who have fathered healthy children. Infertility may, however, be a problem if you are on dialysis. Sperm count usually increases after kidney transplant and the possibility of fathering a child then increases. When you plan a pregnancy, discuss this with your transplant physician who may change your transplant medications to reduce the risk to your unborn child.

Publications that deal with current issues related to kidney failure and treatment, including dialysis, transplantation and adjustment are:

Renalife
Kidney Beginnings
Write to: AAKP
3505 Frontage Road, Suite 315
Tampa, FL 33607
Telephone: 800-749-2257
Website: www.aakp.org

Family Focus
Write to: National Kidney Foundation
30 East 33rd St., 11th floor
New York, NY 10016
Telephone: 800-622-9010
Website: www.kidney.org

National Kidney Foundation of Southern California
Write to: 17100 Ventura Blvd., Suite 222
Encino, CA 91316-4017
Telephone: 800-747-5527
Website: www.kidneysocal.org

Southern California Renal Disease Council, Inc.
ESRD Network 18 (Literature and information)
Write to: 6255 Sunset Blvd., Suite 2211
Hollywood, CA 90028
Telephone: 800-637-4767
e-mail: www.esrdnetwork18.org

Renal Support Network (RSN)
Write to: 1311 N. Maryland Ave.
Glendale, CA 91207
Telephone: 818-543-0896
Website: www.rsnhope.org

How can I meet and talk with other people who have kidney failure?

The American Association of Kidney Patients (AAKP) is an organization of patients for patients. The purpose of AAKP is to promote the welfare of kidney patients through education, and advocacy. Although the national office is located in Florida, there are local chapters in many parts or the United States. These chapters offer educational meetings and social activities that bring patients and families together. For more information on the AAKP and the closest chapter, contact AAKP at 800/749-2257, through e-mail at info@aakp.org, or visit their website at www.aakp.org.

Some National Kidney Foundation affiliates also offer educational meetings for people with kidney failure. For more information on the National Kidney Foundation meetings, contact the local National Kidney Foundation affiliate.

Where can I find help?

If you or your family need help to adjust and cope with kidney failure, you should talk to a social worker. A social worker is a valuable resource person and can help you and your family make the adjustments to kidney disease and treatment. The National Kidney Foundation affiliate and AAKP can also assist with finding help.

Should I seek counseling?

A social worker has the necessary skills and training in counseling and family therapy. If you think that counseling for you and or your family members is needed, you should talk with a social worker. This professional member of the medical team can help determine if counseling can benefit you or members of your family. Discussions with the social worker are confidential.

Unfortunately, many people still believe that kidney failure is terminal, or that people with kidney failure must stay in a hospital bed, attached to a kidney machine, for 24 hours a day. A patient may start dialysis treatment, as many people do, with these beliefs. The fear and anxiety caused by expecting dialysis to be all of the horrible things you have heard and read about can cause difficulty in adjustment. The National Kidney Foundation and its affiliates work with the print and broadcast media to educate the public about the realities of dialysis and kidney failure, including the fact that people who require dialysis treatment can live reasonably normal lives, have friends, work, get married, raise a family and be happy.

How much will what I read and hear affect my adjustment?

The best way to deal with these beliefs and myths about dialysis is for you to meet and talk with other people who are undergoing treatment for kidney failure and with the physician, nurses, social workers and dietitians of your renal center.

A social worker can provide help in counseling services and resource and referral services. Examples of problems that may benefit from counseling services are depression and anxiety, marital and family stress, sexual concerns and concerns about death and dying. Examples of the need for resource and referral services may include inability to pay for the cost of dialysis and transplantation, hospital bills, drugs and doctor bills; lack of transportation for travel to and from dialysis treatments; and loss of employment. A social worker also functions as a patient advocate and is available to help with concerns you may have about treatment. They work as a team member with the other staff in helping you adjust to your illness.

What can the social worker do to help?

Rehabilitation, when the term is applied to someone who has become ill with a chronic medical condition,

What is rehabilitation?

can mean restoring health, positive outlook, meaningful personal relationships, and rewarding activity. Vocational rehabilitation can mean restoring a patient to gainful or useful activities, including housework, childcare, and part-time or full-time work.

Do all people with kidney failure need rehabilitation?

Yes. Some degree of rehabilitation is required for all people undergoing treatment for kidney failure. Restoring health, establishing a positive outlook, maintaining meaningful personal relationships, and pursuing rewarding activities is part of a patient's entire adjustment process. The goal of the medical team at the dialysis unit is to rehabilitate a patient. Whether or not you require vocational rehabilitation depends on your physical health, prior occupation or ability and motivation to find a job.

Can I continue to work?

Most people with kidney failure can return to gainful or useful activities. It helps to have an understanding employer who accepts the fact that your life may be somewhat unstable during the initial adjustment to dialysis and that you may have to take off a few days now and then. In some cases, the type of work that you did prior to kidney disease may be too physically demanding to continue. If you have concerns about your type of work, you should talk to a physician.

Will I have problems finding a job?

The Americans with Disabilities Act of 1990 serves as a protection from discrimination in hiring and employment for people with disabilities. Although people with renal failure may function very well, their need for dialysis treatment may qualify them as disabled for the purposes of this protection. Employers are required to provide "reasonable accommodation" to an employee to enable them to perform their work responsibilities. You must still be able to perform the requirements of the position, but may be able to be accommodated through flexible hours, privacy for fluid exchanges for peritoneal dialysis patients, or other adaptations to the environment that may enable you to continue working.

If you are applying for a new job, a potential employer may not ask you about your health status. You may be asked about your ability to perform the job you are applying for, and a medical examination may be required only if the examination is required for all potential employees in similar positions. The examination must be related to your job.

If you feel that your employment rights may have been violated or that you are being discriminated against because of your health issues, phone the Equal Employment Opportunity Commission at 800-669-4000 or look in your local telephone directory to locate the nearest office. They can help you determine if you should file a charge of discrimination. You do not need a lawyer, although some people elect to retain one.

Employers, as well as the general public, need to be educated to the fact that people receiving dialysis treatment or after kidney transplant can be restored to full productivity. The myths of dialysis disability exist and need to be dealt with. People with kidney failure qualify as disabled under the Americans with Disabilities Act (ADA), which forbids discrimination in hiring prospective employees because of a physical handicap. As is the case with all individuals, however, finding the right job can be a matter of luck, timing and persistence. Sometimes, the biggest stumbling block to finding work is scheduled daytime dialysis treatments. A patient may request a transfer to the evening shift or to another facility that offers late afternoon or evening shifts, or consider peritoneal dialysis that can be performed independently and/or overnight.

Where can I find more information on vocational rehabilitation?

If you are having trouble finding a job or find that you cannot return to the type of work you were doing prior to kidney failure, you may want to seek vocational rehabilitation. For more information, you can contact a social worker or the state Department of Vocational Rehabilitation.

Do I have any rights as a patient?

Yes. Included in the rules and regulations of Public Law 92-603, or the kidney disease provisions of the federal Medicare program, patients or consumers do have rights as well as responsibilities. The rights and responsibilities as a patient are stated in the Federal Register, Volume 41, Number 108, adopted Thursday, June 3, 1976, and are presented, in part, as follows:

The governing body of the ESRD facility adopts written policies regarding the rights and responsibilities of patients and, through the chief executive officer, is responsible for development of, and adherence to, procedures implementing such policies. These policies and procedures are made available to patients and any guardians, next-of-kin, sponsoring agency(ies), representative payees and the public. The staff of the facility is trained and involved in the execution of such policies and procedures. The patients' rights, policies and procedures ensure at least the following:

1. Standard: informed patients. All patients in the facility:
> (a) Are fully informed of these rights and responsibilities, and of all rules and regulations governing patient conduct and responsibilities;

(b) Are fully informed of services available in the facility and of related charges, including any charges for services not covered under title XVIII of the Social Security Act.

(c) Are fully informed by a physician of their medical condition unless medically contraindicated (as documented in their medical records).

2. Standard: participating in planning. All patients treated in the facility:

(a) Are afforded the opportunity to participate in the planning of their medical treatment and to refuse to participate in experimental research;

(b) Are transferred or discharged only for medical reasons, for a patient's welfare or that of other patients, or for nonpayment of fees (except as prohibited by Title XVIII of the Social Security Act), and are given advance notice to ensure orderly transfer or discharge.

3. Standard: respect and dignity. All patients are treated with consideration, respect and full recognition of their individuality and personal needs, including the need for privacy in treatment. Provision is made for translators, where a significant number of patients experience language barriers.

4. Standard: confidentiality. All patients are ensured confidential treatment of their personal and medical records, and may approve or refuse release of such records to any individual outside the facility, except in case of their transfer to another health care institution or as required by federal, state or local law and the secretary for proper administration of the program.

5. Standard: grievance mechanism. All patients are encouraged and assisted to understand and exercise their rights. Grievances and recommended changes in

policies and services may be addressed to facility staff, administration, the Network Council and agencies or regulatory bodies with jurisdiction over the facility, through any representative of a patient's choice, without restraint or interference and without fear of discrimination or reprisal.

How can I help in my own adjustment and rehabilitation? You can educate yourself about kidney failure and treatment. In order to do well with your chronic kidney disease it is important to work closely with your treatment team and report any unusual symptoms or problems that occur. Taking your medications as prescribed and following your diet will help keep you healthy. It is also important to maintain meaningful personal relationships, communicate with your family and friends, participate in rewarding activities, set personal goals, maintain a feeling of self-worth and self-esteem and continue to live your life in the best way you can in spite of kidney failure and its treatment. Your life can continue to be full and satisfying. Your positive attitude can have a profound impact on your adjustment to life with kidney disease.

Which employers are affected by the ADA? All public and private employers who employ 25 or more people for more than 20 weeks in the current or preceding year are included as of July 26, 1992. As of July 26, 1994, all employers employing 15 or more people for more than 20 weeks in the current or preceding year are covered. The United States government, Indian tribes and private membership clubs are not covered; however, the United States government provides similar rights under the Rehabilitation Act of 1993 (29 U.S.C. 706).

Financial Information and Other Resources

What are the costs of treatment for chronic kidney failure?

Currently, the average cost per person for hemodialysis is approximately $65,000 per year. The average cost for kidney transplant surgery without complications is $47,000 in the United States. The federal government and some state programs provide financial assistance to help pay for the costs of treatment for kidney failure. Further information about financial assistance through the federal government is provided in this chapter.

Contact the National Kidney Foundation affiliate for information about federal assistance as well as for information on programs supported by your state.

How can Medicare help?

If a patient qualifies, the Medicare kidney disease provisions cover 80% to 100% of medical and hospital charges. For example, one of the benefits of Medicare is the coverage of EPO when given in a dialysis facility. However, Medicare benefits are limited if the services are also covered by an employer group health plan. These limitations are explained later in this chapter under, "What if a patient has other medical insurance?"

Am I eligible for the kidney disease provisions of Medicare?

You are eligible for benefits under the kidney disease provisions of Medicare if you have kidney failure and are receiving dialysis or have a transplant and meet one of the following qualifications:
- You are fully or currently insured under Social Security or are entitled to a monthly Social Security or Railroad Retirement benefit
- You are the spouse or dependent child of such an individual

If you are over 65 years of age, you may <u>also</u> qualify under the regular Medicare provisions for older people.

Eligibility is not based on age or whether a person is currently working or unable to work.

What are the kidney disease provisions of Medicare? The 1972 kidney disease provisions of Medicare or Public Law 92-603 were effective July 1, 1973. Since then, amendments have been made to expand the program, including the 1978 provision of Public Law 95-292, which were effective October 1, 1978, and the Omnibus Budget Reconciliation Act of 1981, Public Law 97-35, enacted August 13, 1981. The Omnibus Budget Act of 1990 has expanded Medicare coverage of self-administered EPO for home dialysis patients effective 1991; while the Omnibus Reconciliation Act of 1993 (OBRA '93) extends immunosuppressant coverage from one year to three years. The most recent addition to Medicare is the introduction of Part D, the Prescription Drug Benefit which allows seniors and the disabled to obtain subsidized drug coverage.

These Medicare benefits consist of two types of insurance: Part A, or hospital insurance, Part B, or medical insurance, as well as Part D, the prescription drug benefit. Almost everyone who is eligible for Medicare is covered by hospital insurance without paying any monthly premium. Hospital insurance covers medically necessary inpatient hospital care and, under certain conditions, medically necessary post-hospital inpatient care in a skilled nursing facility, and home health care provided by a home health agency. The hospital insurance part of Medicare, for example, helps pay for an inpatient stay in an approved hospital for kidney transplant surgery. Hospital insurance has an annual deductible, and Medicare payments for services are made directly to the participating facility providing services.

When a person becomes entitled to Medicare hospital insurance because of chronic kidney failure they are also enrolled for medical insurance or Part B of Medicare. Although they do not have to take this part of Medicare, most of the services and supplies required by chronic kidney failure are covered only by the medical insurance and not by the hospital insurance. The monthly premium for medical insurance protection covers physicians' services; outpatient hospital services; outpatient maintenance dialysis treatments in an approved dialysis facility; durable medical equipment for use in the home, such as a dialysis machine; and almost all items necessary for home dialysis, as well as many other health services and supplies. In addition to monthly premium payments, medical insurance also carries a small annual deductible payment and a 20 percent coinsurance liability.

If you are entitled to part A or B of Medicare, you also have the option of signing up for a prescription drug benefit, Medicare Part D, which became effective January 1, 2006. Depending upon where you live, there may be a number of different Part D plans to choose from, each with a specific deductible and premium, and each with a different formulary, or list of medications covered by that plan. The program is designed to provide savings to an individual, however, the decision to enroll must be carefully evaluated based on your current coverage and your individual needs. For example, an individual who currently is enrolled in a health maintenance organization risks losing that coverage if he/she enrolls in plan D. For specific information related to your situation, contact Medicare directly at (800) MEDICARE or visit the Medicare website at www.medicare.gov. Additional resources to help people decide if the plan is better for them than their current plan is Medicare Access for Patients RX at www.maprx.info, the Center for Healthcare Rights at 800-434-0222 and the Medicare Rights Center at www. medicarerights.org.

Do I have to be a certain age to be eligible?

No. The kidney disease provisions of Medicare cover a person regardless of age, if they are eligible.

How can I find out if I am eligible for Medicare benefits?

The law states that you must be a Social Security or Railroad Retirement beneficiary or be "fully or currently" insured in order to be eligible for the kidney disease provisions of Medicare. You are currently insured if you have at least six quarters of coverage during the full 12-quarter period ending with the calendar quarter in which dialysis or a transplant occurs. A patient is fully insured when they have one quarter of coverage under the Social Security program for each year elapsing after 1950 (or after the year the patient attains age 21, if later) to the year in which dialysis or transplant occurs. In no case is more than 40 quarters of coverage required. The spouse or dependent child of an insured individual is also eligible. For more information on eligibility, contact the local Social Security office. A social worker can also assist in determining whether or not you are eligible for Medicare benefits.

When and how do I apply for Medicare benefits?

Most people should apply for Medicare benefits after the diagnosis of chronic kidney failure has been made and shortly after beginning treatment. However, the decision to enroll in Medicare should also be based on your current insurance coverage. If you have an Employer Group Health Plan (EGHP), an HMO plan or a COBRA policy, you may want to delay enrolling in Medicare. Applications can be made in person at your local Social Security Administration office or by telephone. To make a telephone appointment to apply for Medicare, phone (800) 772-1213. A social worker may be able to provide assistance in understanding and completing the necessary forms, as can the Social Security Administration representatives.

Medicare coverage for dialysis treatment starts the end of the third month after a course of dialysis is started. For example, if a person were to begin receiving dialysis treatment on May 22nd and continue treatment through the months of June and July, the Medicare coverage would begin August 1st. The purpose of the waiting period is to establish whether or not they have chronic kidney failure rather than acute kidney failure which often is reversible. The Government refers to the waiting period as a qualifying period. This waiting period may be eliminated depending on the type of treatment chosen, and if this decision is made during the first three months after treatment begins. For more information on eliminating the waiting period, you should talk to a social worker. (See Chapter 3).

What is the waiting period?

Part B medical insurance helps pay for outpatient maintenance dialysis treatments in any approved dialysis facility, including the costs of laboratory tests, equipment, supplies and other services associated with treatment. Charges for maintenance dialysis vary from one approved facility to another. Medicare pays the facility based on a per treatment rate set in advance. This rate is known as the composite rate. Medicare pays 80 percent of the composite rate less any part of the Part B deductible the patient has not met. You are responsible for any unmet Part B deductible plus the remaining 20 percent of the composite rate. The facility may never charge more than the unmet Part B deductible plus 20 percent of its Medicare composite rate.

What costs in dialysis are covered by Medicare?

Physicians' services are also covered while you are receiving dialysis treatment. Medicare pays for these services through a monthly capitation payment. This amount is paid regardless of whether a patient dialyzes as an outpatient in a dialysis facility, or at home. Under this method, Medicare pays 80 percent of a physician's monthly payment less any unmet Part B deductible. A patient pays any unmet Part B deductible plus the remaining 20 percent of the monthly payment. If a physician accepts assignment, Medicare pays them directly, and you may not be charged more than the unmet Part B deductible plus 20 percent of the monthly payment. (Assignment means that a physician accepts the amount approved by Medicare as the total payment.) If a physician does not accept assignment, you receive the doctor's payment directly and there is no limit on the amount that may be charged by the physician.

If you are admitted to a hospital because your medical condition requires the availability of other specialized hospital services on an inpatient basis, the maintenance dialysis treatments would be covered by hospital insurance, Part A, as part of the costs of the covered inpatient hospital stay. While you are in the hospital, a physician may choose to be paid for each individual service they provide. In this case, a physician receives a prorated portion of the monthly capitation payment, reduced in proportion to the number of days you are hospitalized.

What are the Medicare benefits for self-care dialysis? If people participate in a self-care training program within the first three months after treatment begins with the intention of doing self-care (home) dialysis, Medicare benefits start during the month the self-care training begins.

Is home dialysis covered by Medicare? Yes. In addition to eliminating the waiting period, if you begin training for self-care or home dialysis within the first thee months after treatment begins, Medicare covers home dialysis equipment, all necessary supplies, and a wide range of home support services. Home dialysis includes home hemodialysis, continuous ambulatory peritoneal dialysis (CAPD), continuous cycling peritoneal dialysis (CCPD) and home intermittent peritoneal dialysis (IPD). Medicare medical insurance covers rental or purchase of the dialysis equipment for home use including delivery and installation service charges. If you stop using your home dialysis equipment temporarily, for example, because you are traveling or are hospitalized, medical insurance continues payment for the equipment for up to three months after the month in which you last used it. Medicare, through the medical insurance, covers all supplies necessary to perform home dialysis, including disposable items, such as alcohol wipes, sterile drapes, rubber gloves, forceps, scissors and topical anesthetics. Drugs cannot be covered except for heparin, the heparin antidote and topical anesthetics. The medical insurance also covers periodic support services furnished by a hospital or facility, which may be necessary to assist people who remain on home dialysis. Such support services may include visits by trained hospital or facility personnel to periodically monitor their dialysis and to assist in emergencies when necessary. In addition, services of a qualified facility or hospital personnel are covered to help with the installation and maintenance of the dialysis equipment. After the annual deductible is paid, Medicare pays 80 percent of all costs and services related to home dialysis treatment. Medicare does not pay for a home helper to assist with dialysis at home.

How does Medicare pay for home dialysis?

There are two payment options to choose from if a person dialyzes at home: Method I or Method II. To make a choice, a person completes the Beneficiary Selection Form HCFA-382, signs it and returns it to the facility supervising their care. The decision to select either Method I or Method II is a personal choice depending upon one's preference to work directly with Medicare or to have the dialysis facility handle the arrangements. Once a patient makes an initial choice, he or she must continue under that option until the end of the year. A patient can change from one Method to the other at any time by filing a new Form 382, but the change does not go into effect until the following January 1. It is important to remember that choosing Method I or Method II does not in any way prevent a patient from returning to treatment in a center, selecting another kind of treatment or choosing to associate with another facility. The two methods are:

Method I: The Composite Rate
Method II: Dealing Directly with Medicare

Method I: The Composite Rate

If you choose Method I, the dialysis facility is responsible for providing all services, equipment and supplies necessary for home dialysis. Medicare pays the facility directly for these items and services at a predetermined composite rate. Under this arrangement, you are responsible for paying the annual deductible and the 20 percent coinsurance on the Medicare rate to the facility.

Method II: Dealing Directly with Medicare

If you choose Method II, you receive payment directly from Medicare for covered home dialysis equipment and supplies. Under this arrangement, you must obtain these items directly from a supplier and are responsible for paying the supplier. However, if you choose to obtain the home dialysis equipment and supplies from a facility, Medicare pays the facility directly. Whether people obtain their items from a supplier or from a facility, they are responsible for any unmet part of the annual deductible and for 20 percent coinsurance of the approved charges for these items.

Under both Methods, a person must receive home dialysis support services from a facility, for which Medicare pays the facility directly.

Yes. Peritoneal dialysis treatment in a hospital or dialysis facility has the same coverage as hemodialysis in a hospital or facility. Continuous ambulatory peritoneal dialysis (CAPD), continuous cycling peritoneal dialysis (CCPD) and home intermittent peritoneal dialysis (IPD) are covered with the same benefits as home hemodialysis.

Is peritoneal dialysis covered by Medicare?

The waiting period for Medicare benefits is waived if a person receives a kidney transplant during the waiting period. As a transplant recipient, they are eligible for Medicare Part A and Part B benefits including coverage of costs related to:

What are the Medicare benefits for kidney transplantation?

- hospital, nursing, laboratory tests and tissue typing
- surgeon and related costs of surgery
- intensive care and post-surgical costs
- subsequent follow-up after transplantation
- routine costs associated with the retrieval of a donor kidney, including living related, living unrelated and deceased donors

Medicare's hospital insurance provides 100 percent of the hospital stay and transplant operation after the annual deductible is paid. Medicare's medical insurance covers 90 percent of the cost associated with follow-up physician visits and care. Eighty percent of immunosuppressant drug expenses are covered for one year following transplantation. The Omnibus Reconciliation Act of 1993 (OBRA '93) extended immunosuppressant coverage from one year to three years for those receiving transplants after 1995. After transplantation, Medicare coverage continues for an additional 36 months and may be extended if you are disabled or unable to work. If the transplanted kidney is rejected or lost during this time, your return to dialysis is covered immediately.

Who pays for the living related donor's medical costs?

Medicare covers the full cost of medical services for a living related donor, including coinsurance and deductibles.

What if I have other medical insurance?

If there is other medical insurance, Medicare pays to the limit of its liability and the supplementary insurer generally pays that portion of the balance remaining unpaid. There is an exception, however, if the other insurance is an employer group health plan. In that case, Medicare pays only secondary benefits for a period of up to 30 months. During this period, the employer plan pays first for dialysis and other health services. If the employer plan pays less than the amount of the provider's cost or charge, Medicare may make secondary payment to supplement the amount paid by the employer plan. At the end of the 30-month period, Medicare pays primary benefits.

Do I have to pay anything when receiving primary Medicare benefits?

Yes. You must pay the Part A hospital insurance deductible at the start of each benefit period of hospitalization as well as the Part B medical insurance annual deductible and monthly premium. You are responsible for the 20 percent coinsurance that is not covered by Part B medical insurance and all costs not covered under either plan. It may be helpful for you to talk with a social worker or dialysis unit administrator about the 20 percent coinsurance or about any other financial concerns. This can clarify any misunderstanding you have about your financial responsibilities.

What happens if I receive a Medicare check?

If you receive a check directly from Medicare, it is intended to pay the provider of treatment, unless you have already paid for these services. In addition, the provider needs the portion attached to the Medicare check for billing purposes.

The Social Security Administration office has more information on the kidney disease provisions of Medicare as do most social workers in dialysis units. A free publication entitled Medicare Coverage of Kidney Dialysis and Kidney Transplant Services is available at the Social Security Administration office. There is also a great deal of information available on the internet and at www.medicare.gov.

To whom can I talk for more information about Medicare benefits?

Medicaid (MediCal in California) is a federal state-supported program to pay for health care for needy and low-income residents. Medicaid benefits vary from state to state.

What is Medicaid?

Medicare eligibility is based on a diagnosis of chronic kidney failure and on the number of quarters paid into a person's Social Security account. Eligibility for Medicaid is based on a diagnosis of chronic kidney failure and on financial need.

What is the difference between Medicare and Medicaid?

You cannot earn more than a specified annual income to be eligible for Medicaid; this income varies from one state to another. To determine Medicaid eligibility, you should contact the county welfare department in your community. A social worker can assist in referring you to the proper Department of Public Social Service office or the Social Security office for eligibility information. Pamphlets regarding Medicare may be available from a social worker or the National Kidney Foundation affiliate in your area and at the Social Security Administration office.

How can I find out if I am eligible for Medicaid?

Yes. A partial list with a brief description has been included below. For more information on federal programs and eligibility, you should talk with a social worker.

Are there other federal programs that can help?

Veterans Administration. If you are a veteran and if the disease is service-connected, you are eligible for treatment at a VA hospital. If you do not have service-connected kidney disease, you may still be eligible for treatment at a VA hospital if the VA hospital has room in its program and chooses to provide treatment. For more information on eligibility, contact the Veterans Administration.

Social Security Disability Insurance. Social Security Disability Insurance provides a source of income for those who qualify for benefits. Qualifications include two factors: how old you are in relation to how long you have worked and the extent of your physical limitations. To qualify, you must be unable to participate in "substantial gainful activity" for a period of at least 12 months. Substantial gainful activity means that you cannot work; this must be documented by a physician's statement or by a medical facility. The first five months are not covered by disability insurance; payments begin the sixth month from the date of onset of disability. The local Social Security Administration office can provide more information.

Supplemental Security Income (SSI). If you are disabled, blind or over 65, you may be eligible to receive SSI if you meet financial eligibility criteria. Many people apply for SSI while they are awaiting their Social Security Disability. You should apply for SSI at the Social Security Administration office. It may take several months for SSI benefits to be approved.

Veterans Pensions. If you are a veteran, you may be eligible for a pension from the Veterans Administration if your income is low.

Who can help me with my finances? A social worker can provide you with more information on financial assistance for medical expenses as well as everyday living expenses. The National Kidney Foundation affiliate can also assist you in identifying resources for financial assistance.

Organizations that provide limited financial support include some affiliates of the National Kidney Foundation, the American Association of Kidney Patients (AAKP) 800-749-2257, and the American Kidney Fund 800-638-8299.

What organizations provide financial help?

The National Kidney Foundation is the national voluntary health agency that strives to prevent kidney and urinary tract diseases and that provides services to people living with kidney disease. It supports research, public and professional education, patient and community services and public policy. The National Kidney Foundation has affiliates throughout the nation, with professional staff to service the community. Each affiliate is governed by a voluntary board of directors and offers programs and services to meet the needs of its community. For more information on the National Kidney Foundation and the location of the closest affiliate, contact: National Kidney Foundation, 30 East 33rd St. 11th floor, New York, NY 10016; or call toll free 800-622-9010; or www.kidney. org. In Southern California, contact: National Kidney Foundation of Southern California, 17100 Ventura Blvd., Suite 222, Encino, CA 91316-4017; or call toll free 800-747-5527; or www.kidneysocal.org.

What is the National Kidney Foundation?

The National Kidney Foundation and its affiliates maintain information and referral services that may provide information on financial eligibility, resources and referral to other agencies that provide direct financial assistance. (Some affiliates do provide direct financial assistance.) For more information on financial assistance and services,

What can the National Kidney Foundation do to help?

contact the National Kidney Foundation affiliate in your local area.

When should I call the National Kidney Foundation?

Most affiliates of the National Kidney Foundation maintain an information and referral service during regular business hours. This service is available to any member of the community in need of information and/or referral services relating to kidney disease and treatment. Although the Foundation cannot give medical advice, it can provide written and/or verbal information on kidney disease, treatments, availability of medical services and financial assistance.

What does the National Kidney Foundation do for people with kidney disease?

National Kidney Foundation affiliates vary in the types of the programs and services they offer. In addition to maintaining an information and referral service for people with kidney disease and their families, many affiliates offer free literature on kidney diseases and methods of treatment, as well as a variety of other valuable services. For more information on the types of service offered, contact your local National Kidney Foundation affiliate.

Is the National Kidney Foundation involved in legislation and advocacy for people with kidney disease?

Yes. The National Kidney Foundation and its affiliates have supported and continue to support legislation on both a federal and state level, advocating increased benefits and support for people living with kidney and urinary tract disease and kidney failure. The National Kidney Foundation was very instrumental in passing the federal legislation, which, in 1973, enabled kidney patients to receive Medicare benefits.

Does the National Kidney Foundation support research?

Yes. The National Kidney Foundation and its affiliates have funded millions of dollars for research support to investigate the causes, prevention and treatment of kidney and urinary tract diseases and kidney failure, improvement of dialysis results, increased success rates for kidney transplantation and alternative methods of treatment for kidney failure.

In addition to services directed to people with kidney disease, the National Kidney Foundation and its affiliates provide professional education, public education and promotion of organ donation. Some affiliates sponsor an early detection or screening program to test for asymptomatic urinary tract infections and undiagnosed high blood pressure. The National Kidney Foundation has convened several panels of kidney disease professionals to evaluate and establish guidelines for providing patients with the very highest quality of care. These guidelines are called K/DOQI guidelines and these are continually undergoing review and revision as new research results become available.

What other services does the National Kidney Foundation provide?

The American Association of Kidney Patients (AAKP) is a voluntary patient organization dedicated to helping renal patients and their families deal with kidney disease through a variety of publications, educational conferences and legislative education. Chapters of AAKP are active in a variety of educational and social events and supportive programs designed to support patients' and families' ability to participate in planning and managing their treatment and to improve public programs that help kidney patients meet their financial and personal needs, as well as to participate in public policy issues. For more information about AAKP and the location of local chapters, call 800-749-2257 or go to their website at www.aakp.org.

What aid does the American Association of Kidney Patients (AAKP) give?

The William B. Dessner Memorial Fund, Inc. provides modest emergency financial aid to kidney dialysis and transplant patients at the request of their social workers. For more information, write to: The William B. Dessner Memorial Fund, Inc., 2200 Colorado Avenue, Ste. 503, Santa Monica, CA 90404.

What aid does the William B. Dessner Memorial Fund, Inc. give?

Can the American Kidney Fund help? The American Kidney Fund may provide direct financial assistance to people with kidney disease, including dialysis and transplant patients. Grants are based on the nature of the requirement, on urgency and on the availability of funds. For further information, on eligibility and applications, contact: American Kidney Fund, 6110 Executive Blvd., Rockville, MD 20852. Call toll free 800-638-8299 or www.kidneyfund.org.

What is the Network Council? Public Law 95-292 or the 1978 provisions of the Medicare program established regional "networks" for the coordination and review of dialysis and transplant facilities and programs. Each network covers an area within the United States without regard to state lines. Within each network is a coordinating council composed of individuals knowledgeable about kidney failure and treatment programs. Network offices also have paid staff members. All networks consist of a Network Coordinating Council and Medical Review Board. The function of the Network Coordinating Council, along with the Medical Review Board, is to assess the appropriateness of patient care and to assure the highest possible quality of medical care. At least one patient representative shall serve on each council. The other members of the coordinating council include physicians and health personnel involved in the care of kidney patients. For more information on the function of the coordinating council and Medical Review Board, contact the local National Kidney Foundation affiliate.

Are there any other organizations that provide services? Yes. The Polycystic Kidney Disease Foundation was formed for people with polycystic kidney disease and their families. This organization sponsors research and distributes information to patients and medical professionals. For more information, contact: Polycystic Kidney Disease Foundation, 9221 Ward Parkway, Suite 400, Kansas City, MO 64106, or go to their website at www.pkdcure.org.

The Renal Support Network (RSN) is a nonprofit, patient-focused, patient-run organization established in 1993 to provide non-medical services to those affected by chronic kidney disease (CKD). RSN strives to help patients develop their personal coping skills, special talents, and employability by educating and empowering them (and their family members) to take control of the course and management of the disease. A vital role of RSN is to provide lawmakers and policy makers with the patients' perspective on the needs and capabilities of people with CKD. For more information, contact The Renal Support Network, 1311 N. Maryland Avenue, Glendale, CA 91207, or go to their website at www.rsnhope.org for more information.

Life Options is a program of research, research-based education and outreach that helps people live long and well with kidney disease. A national panel of doctors, researchers patients, nurses, social workers, dietitians and ESRD Network directors review all Life Options materials and help guide research. For more information, contact Life Options c/o Medical Education Institute, Inc., 414 D'Onofrio Drive, Suite 200, Madison, WI 53719, or go to their website at www.lifeoptions.org.

Can I still travel if I require dialysis treatment?

Yes. There are many dialysis centers within the United States and internationally that accept traveling or transient people. Prior arrangements are necessary and physician approval is advised. Medicare, however, will not pay for services outside the United States.

How do I make the necessary arrangements to travel? Who can help?

Dialysis units vary in their ability to assist in travel dialysis planning. The charge nurse on the dialysis unit, the primary nurse (the one who assists in treatment), or a social worker may be able to help you with the necessary paperwork and arrangements. The dialysis unit will also be asked to supply the visiting unit with individual dialysis information. If you have determined, after talking to the dialysis staff that you have primary responsibility for making the arrangements, you should contact the dialysis center at the vacation spot. Whether you write or call, you should do the following:

1. State your name, city and state.
2. Inform the unit about where you dialyze regularly, how often and the length of each treatment.
3. Specify if you are hepatitis positive or negative and ask if the unit accepts people who are positive, negative, or both. If the unit accepts positive people for example, and you are negative, you should ask to be referred to a hepatitis negative unit in the area, or to a unit that separates the positive and negative people to prevent the spread of infection. It is important that you talk to the dialysis physician about the unit's policy before making any travel arrangements.
4. Inform the unit how long you wish to dialyze there and on what dates.

What kind of information is requested by other dialysis centers?

1. **HCFA 2728:** This is the Medicare Chronic Renal Disease (CRD) Medical Evidence Report describing a person's current medical status, in codeable terms for computer storage. It is used to indicate Medicare eligibility when the visiting dialysis facility bills Medicare for treatments. Ask for a photocopy of this form from the business office of the hospital or center where you normally dialyze.
2. **Physician's Summary:** This is a medical summary of the current situation and is to be completed by the dialysis physician. It is requested to give the visiting dialysis unit an idea of a person's diagnosis, previous medical treatment and current status.
3. **Patient Information Sheet:** This sheet describes the dialysis treatments in terms of length of treatments, dialysis

frequency, type of dialyzer used, medications, current lab values, any known complications or allergies, and insurance information. Usually, the charge nurse or primary nurse assists you in completing this form.

4. **Hepatitis B Antigen Test:** This blood test verifies the hepatitis factor. Usually a person sends verification of their hepatitis status to the distant unit along with the other required dialysis information. Approximately 10 days prior to your trip, another Hepatitis B surface Antigen should be drawn; the original should be forwarded to the distant unit and a copy should be hand-carried.

How do I find a dialysis unit at my vacation spot?

Many dialysis units, especially those in areas of high tourist demand, such as Hawaii, California, Arizona and Florida, need two or three months notice of your visit, particularly if you plan to stay longer than one or two weeks. If you plan to travel during a holiday season, you should contact the unit six months in advance. Since the units operate on a first-come, first-served basis, it is advisable to make a request as early as possible. To determine where to dialyze in a travel spot, you should first check with the charge nurse or a social worker in your dialysis unit for a listing of dialysis units throughout the country. You can research dialysis units on the internet at www.medicare.gov/dialysis and look under "Dialysis Facility Compare" to find a unit near your destination. Another way to locate dialysis units is at www.dialysisfinder.com, and to locate units outside of the United States, through www.globaldialysis.com. Your dialysis unit may have their own travel service to assist you in the process of locating a unit near your vacation destination.

Will Medicare pay for my treatment when I travel?

Yes. If you are currently receiving Medicare benefits, these same benefits apply toward treatment at a vacation spot within the United States. At the time you contact the dialysis unit requesting visiting dialysis, you should ask them to clarify the payment procedure. The method of payment for dialysis treatment varies from unit to unit. All dialysis units are required by law to bill Medicare for 80 percent of their allowable payment rate. Some dialysis units, particularly those located in hospitals that have large business offices, bill the supplementary insurance carrier for the remaining 20 percent. However, many units affiliated with hospitals, but not necessarily located in hospitals, ask you to pay the remaining 20 percent in cash. You should take the insurance forms from the supplemental carrier on the trip and have them filled out by the unit personnel so that there is no delay in your insurance company's reimbursement.

If you have Medicare coverage, parts A and B, and do not have a supplemental insurance policy to pick up the remaining 20 percent of your dialysis costs, you should inquire at the hospital business office to see how the 20 percent is currently being paid. If you are receiving Medicaid only and wish to travel, it is important for you to discuss this with a social worker since prior approval may be necessary before receiving guest dialysis out-of-state.

Is there anything else I should know about making travel plans?

Yes. Normally, dialysis patients from a unit in which hepatitis is present can best be accommodated by a comparable unit. While this factor may require careful planning and unit coordination and support, it is wise to be persistent in checking all available dialysis units in your desired area. Some large dialysis units in metropolitan areas may be more flexible, since they have established separate hepatitis negative and hepatitis positive dialysis units. You should talk with their dialysis physician and charge nurse regarding policy for dialysis in their unit and follow that policy.

When you arrive in the area that you are visiting, you

should get settled, then call the dialysis unit to confirm the dialysis reservation and recheck the reporting time for the dialysis treatment.

Yes. There are travel agencies that assist in scheduling dialysis. Some of these agencies coordinate cruises and provide treatment during the cruise. For more information, contact the local National Kidney Foundation affiliate.

Are there any travel agencies that specialize in travel arrangements for people on dialysis?

Yes. There are many books available.

Highly recommended:

Understanding Your New Life With Dialysis, Fourth edition, by Edith T. Oberley, M.A., and Terry D. Oberley, M.D., Ph.D. Dr. Terry Oberley is currently receiving dialysis treatment and has been for many years. This book describes his adjustment to kidney failure and dialysis, and provides a variety of useful information on kidney failure and treatment. Write to Charles C. Thomas, 2600 South First St., Springfield, IL 62617 or go the website at www. ccthomas.com.

Ask a physician or social worker for the titles of other books on kidney failure and treatment.

Are there any books available to give me more information about kidney failure and treatment?

Chapter Nine

Research and Kidney Failure

Is research being done on kidney failure?

Yes. Ongoing research is being done in the United States to:
- Better understand the causes of kidney diseases and kidney failure
- Develop new ways to treat and prevent kidney diseases and kidney failure
- Improve dialysis therapies
- Increase success rates for kidney transplantation
- Find alternative treatment methods for treating kidney failure

What are some of the more important research accomplishments?

As a result of intensive research and advances in technology, the treatment of kidney failure has changed and expanded. Many advances have made it possible for people with kidney failure to live longer and with fewer complications. This includes:
- The use of recombinant erythropoietin to treat the anemia of chronic kidney failure. Erythropoietin has reduced the need for blood transfusions and has improved the exercise endurance and feeling of well-being of people with kidney failure. A new formulation of erythropoietin lasts longer in the body and can be injected less frequently than the old version. However both versions are effective in improving the blood count and improving patient energy and well-being
- A better understanding of the immunology of transplantation that has led to the ongoing development of new medications and tissue typing techniques to prevent the rejection of transplanted kidneys
- The effective use of a new medication called cinacalcet, for the treatment of a common form of bone disease that occurs with kidney failure
- The development of new medications with fewer side-effects to bind phosphorus that comes from

the diet, which enhances bone health

- The continued improvement of peritoneal dialysis so that the risk of infection has been significantly reduced
- The aggressive use of medications known as ACE inhibitors and angiotensin receptor blockers (or ARBs) which inhibit the hormone angiotensin II, for the purpose of slowing the progression of kidney disease due to diabetes and other causes

Are there any other recent research developments?

Yes. There have been several recent research developments that have led to new ways of preventing kidney failure and treating people with kidney failure.

The development of new and more effective antihypertensive (high blood pressure) medications now offers more treatment options for people with hypertension. Hypertension remains a major cause of kidney failure.

Studies are being done to find out if hemodialysis is better tolerated and more effective if given in a different way than the usual three times a week schedule. Some data suggest that dialysis given slowly overnight (eg. 8 hour sessions), given for 2 to 2 ½ hours a day 6 days a week, or even done at home for 2 – 2 ½ hours 5-7 times a week, helps patients feel better, lowers blood pressure without blood pressure medicine, permits for a less restricted diet, enhances well-being, and supports overall longer and healthier lives for people with end stage kidney disease. The development of new CAPD systems has dramatically reduced the incidence of peritonitis, the most common complication of CAPD.

Improvements in the use of immunosuppressive medications in preventing the rejection of kidney transplants and in tissue type matching have increased the success rate of kidney transplantation.

Is there promising research taking place now? Yes. Research centers throughout the United States and the world are doing research in the treatment of people with kidney failure.

Examples of promising research include:

- development of continuous computerized monitoring of hemodialysis treatment to improve the safety and the quality of dialysis

- improving the understanding of the interaction between the blood and hemodialyzer membranes so that even safer and more efficient membranes can be developed

- developing new strategies to prevent heart problems that lead to hospitalizations or death in patients receiving hemodialysis

- developing new ways to reduce the risk of infection in patients receiving dialysis treatments

- development of portable dialysis machines

- treatment of a variety of kidney diseases and conditions that can lead to chronic kidney failure

- development of new immunosuppressives, immunosuppressive strategies and tissue typing techniques to optimize the success rate of kidney transplantation

- development of new ways of preserving donor kidneys for transplantation so that the best possible tissue matching and early function of the transplanted kidney may be achieved

- development of medications that may reverse scarring, so that kidneys that still work but have very advanced disease that were previously thought to be beyond recovery, may potentially improve

- development of new treatment options in the early stages of polycystic kidney disease

Scientific studies exploring the molecular and cell biology and physiology of kidney diseases and kidney failure eventually lead to new ways of preventing and treating kidney failure. Studies on cell culture and animal models for human kidney diseases and kidney failure show important new insights into the many factors that add to the causes and complications of kidney diseases and kidney failure. They have also provided a scientific basis for developing new approaches to preventing and treating kidney failure.

New molecular biological techniques are being applied to the study of kidney diseases with a genetic basis. It offers hope that, in the future, treatment of diseases, such as polycystic kidney disease, will become a reality. Even diseases that are genetically more complex than polycystic kidney disease, such as diabetic kidney disease, are being studied from a genetic point of view. Genetic studies in these "complex" genetic disorders may also lead to new treatments. Advances in our scientific understanding of the molecular and cell biology of kidney transplantation ensure continued improvements in the success, safety and availability of kidney transplantation for people with kidney failure. Although use of some of these scientific advances on patients may be years in the future, new scientific explorations must be encouraged and supported so that present and future generations of people with kidney disease and kidney failure may benefit.

Is there ongoing research that may lead to future advances in the prevention and treatment of kidney diseases and kidney failure?

Research in kidney diseases and kidney failure is being done throughout the world. Many of the top kidney research facilities in the world are located in the United States under the supervision of internationally recognized scientists.

Where is research being done?

Who is paying for the research on kidney failure and treatment?

Most of the funding for research in the United States comes from the federal government through the National Institutes of Health. The second-largest non-commercial source of funding comes from the National Kidney Foundation and its affiliates throughout the United States. Pharmaceutical firms also support research. They test their products so the results can be presented to the Food and Drug Administration, and support basic research that may lead to new treatments.

How can information about the latest kidney research developments be obtained?

There are several magazines that publish information on the latest research developments in kidney disease and kidney failure. One very good source is Renalife, which is published by the American Association of Kidney Patients (AAKP). Contemporary Dialysis and Nephrology (CD&N) publishes the latest scientific research developments. Regional National Kidney Foundation affiliates are also a good resource for this information; anyone can request to be placed on local mailing lists for their newsletters.

Pediatric Kidney Disease

About half of children who require dialysis or a kidney transplant during childhood suffer from a kidney disorder that they were born with. Examples are an obstruction (blockage to the drainage of urine) or abnormally formed, cystic kidneys. Some other common causes of kidney failure in childhood include focal segmental glomerulosclerosis (FSGS), hemolytic-uremic syndrome (HUS), autosomal recessive polycystic kidney disease, vesicoureteral reflux (urine backing up into the kidneys when the child empties his or her bladder), and various kinds of glomerulonephritis.

Which diseases cause kidney failure in children?

In the 0 to 19 year age group there are about 15 new cases of kidney failure per million child population. The incidence also varies by age – 9 per million in 0-4 year olds, 7 per million in 5-9 year olds, 14 per million in 10-14 year olds, and 28 per million in 15-19 year olds. There are currently about 8000 children under age 19 in the United States who are living on dialysis or with a kidney transplant.

How common is kidney failure in childhood?

In children with blockage of the urinary tract or with some other congenital kidney abnormalities, changes might be found during a routine prenatal ultrasound sometime after 14 weeks of the pregnancy. If there is a high risk of kidney abnormalities or if kidneys look abnormal on the screening ultrasound, a more complex ultrasound could be done. The complex ultrasound would be expected to find milder changes. Prenatal ultrasound is a painless, safe procedure.

How early can kidney disease be detected in a child?

In rare instances where the blockage of the urinary system is causing problems with the baby's development, a prenatal surgery to reroute the urine might be recommended. This kind of surgery is only done in very rare instances.

Can anything be done to fix kidney problems before the child is born?

What special problems do children with kidney failure face?

Poor growth is one of the problems that children with kidney disease face, especially children with significantly reduced kidney function at a very early age. Like adults with kidney disease, children with kidney disease often have poor appetites, and lack the proper nutrition to grow well. In addition, the bone disease that goes along with kidney failure interferes with growth.

Can anything be done to improve growth in children with chronic kidney disease?

Children with chronic kidney disease need to have a careful evaluation of their nutritional needs. Their diets must provide enough calories, the right amount of protein, and correct amount of phosphorus to keep the bones healthy and growing. They may also need to take some medication to work against the excess acid that is often in the blood when children have chronic kidney disease. The excess acid in the blood weakens the bones and can lead to poor growth. Blood phosphorus levels must be kept under control. If treatment of all of these abnormalities fail to improve the child's growth, then growth hormone therapy can be prescribed.

What is growth hormone and how does it work?

Growth hormone is a hormone that is made in our bodies, and it promotes growth. It only improves growth in children whose bones are capable of growing. This is usually before children are 14 or 15 years of age. Pharmaceutical companies make human growth hormone. It is approved by the FDA (Food and Drug Administration) for use in children with kidney failure. It needs to be given daily by an injection. Fortunately only a small dose is needed, and the needles used are very small. The growth hormone is given by the child's parent or guardian at home. Older children may learn how to give themselves injections.

Chronic peritoneal dialysis can sometimes be done in small infants weighing as little as 4 pounds. However, infants that small can experience increased complications. Hemodialysis is technically more difficult in small infants than it is in larger children. Hemodialysis in small children is usually done using a catheter instead of with a vascular access (fistula or graft). Chronic dialysis in a very young infant is very demanding on the infant and family. The goal in dialyzing these infants is to keep them healthy and improve their growth until they can get a kidney transplant.

How big does a child need to be to be on dialysis?

Though it sounds surprising, children with kidney failure tend to do better in the long run if they receive a kidney transplant from an adult. To allow space for an adult kidney, the child usually needs to weigh at least 20 or 22 pounds. Some pediatric transplant centers will transplant children as small as 16 or 18 pounds.

How large does a child need to be to get a kidney transplant?

In older children, the transplanted kidney is placed in the same spot as it is in adults, in the groin area. In infants and small children, the kidney is placed in the abdominal cavity. The placement of the kidney in the abdominal cavity is more complicated, so most infants and small children do not start eating as soon after surgery as older children and adults do, and the actual operation takes longer.

Is the kidney transplant placed in the same spot as the adult?

Children usually do very well after transplant with the most dramatic changes seen in the smallest children. Small children tend to show the best improvements in growth, though many children grow very well after transplant. The survival of children and the survival of their kidney transplants are at least as good as the survival in adults after transplantation.

How do children do after a kidney transplant?

What would cause a kidney transplant to fail in a child? Though most kidney transplants last many years, they can lose function for several reasons. Some kidneys may be lost due to the original kidney disease coming back. Some are lost due to slow deterioration from chronic rejection. Some are lost because of toxicity of the anti-rejection medications. Some are lost because children start skipping their immunosuppressive medications. Even a perfectly functioning kidney transplant can be lost many years after the operation if the immunosuppressive medications are stopped or taken irregularly.

What can be done to be sure that children and teenagers take their medications regularly? Children and teenagers need to become partners in the treatment of their kidney disease and kidney transplant as soon as they are old enough to understand what kidney disease is and what all of their medications do. Families and the whole transplant team need to work together on this very important learning process. In addition, children need to assume responsibility for helping with chores at home, and need to play an active role in participating in their educational and career plans.

Diabetes and Kidney Disease

Diabetes is the most common cause of chronic kidney disease in the United States. However, being diabetic does not necessarily mean your kidneys will become damaged. Your kidneys filter waste products from the blood and produce urine. In those susceptible, the persistent high blood sugar damages the tiny blood vessels in the kidneys. Diabetic kidney disease is characterized by the leakage of protein, called albumin, into the urine. Initially, the healthy parts of the kidney are able to compensate for the damaged portions. Over time, more albumin begins to leak into the urine, and the filtering ability of the kidney starts to deteriorate.

How does diabetes affect the kidney?

Yes, there are two major types:

Type I diabetes usually presents in childhood, and makes up 5-10% of cases in the United States. In Type I diabetes, the pancreas is unable to produce insulin, and therefore, insulin injections are required. 20-40% of patients with Type I diabetes develop kidney failure by age 50.

Type II diabetes usually presents in adulthood, after age 45 although its incidence has increased in younger individuals as well. It is the form of diabetes often associated with obesity. In Type II diabetes, the body becomes resistant to the effects of insulin. Many, but not all, Type II diabetics require pills and/or insulin to control their blood sugar.

Are there different forms of diabetes?

There are a variety of tests that can be used to assess your kidney function, and your doctor may perform a combination of blood and urine tests. The amount of protein lost in the urine can be checked with a test called a urinalysis, a simple urine test. Once you are on medications to control the amount of protein in your urine, urinalysis can be repeated regularly to check for improvement. Urinalysis should be performed at least

How can I be tested for diabetic kidney disease?

yearly to check for protein in the urine.

Your doctor may also use a blood test for creatinine. Creatinine is a normal waste product that is produced by working muscles and is cleared out of the blood by the kidneys. When kidney function is reduced, creatinine levels increase. By measuring creatinine, and using a formula that accounts for your age, race, and gender, your doctor can calculate your glomerular filtration rate, or GFR, an index of how well your kidneys are functioning. With this information, your doctor can prescribe appropriate therapies and lifestyle changes for your level of kidney disease.

Can you have diabetic kidney disease and not even know it? Yes. The early phases are characterized by the leakage of very small amounts of albumin into the urine, called microalbuminuria. This phase of the disease is usually free of symptoms. Over time, the filtering ability of the kidneys becomes impaired, but an individual can lose 90% of their kidney function and still remain free of symptoms. By the time you begin to experience symptoms, you may already have advanced kidney failure. Therefore, it's extremely important to see your doctor regularly to have routine tests performed that can pick up kidney disease early.

My doctor told me the diabetes is affecting my kidney. How soon are my kidneys going to fail? There is no set rate of progression to kidney failure, and every individual is different. In general, diabetic kidney disease is a slow process that takes years to develop. Kidney disease usually does not occur within the first 10 years of the development of diabetes. Usually 15-25 years pass before kidney failure occurs. Some patients with diabetes may never develop kidney disease.

Diets should be tailor-made for each individual patient by working with a dietician. A dietician can create a diet for you based on your diabetes control, your stage of kidney disease, and the presence or absence of any other medical conditions (such as high blood pressure or heart disease).

Patients with more advanced kidney disease will need to watch their intake of certain substances such as potassium (found in oranges, tomatoes, and bananas, among many other foods) and phosphorus (found in colas and dairy products) to avoid toxic levels. These changes will be discussed with you by your doctor and dietician.

What should my diet be?

The amount of protein that should be in your diet remains controversial among experts, and should be tailored for individual patients by their doctor and dietician. However, research has shown that excessive protein in the diet may be harmful for patients with kidney disease. For patients with near-normal kidney function, a diet consistent with the U.S. RDA (recommended daily allowance) recommendations for protein intake appears to be acceptable. A high-protein diet should be avoided. For people whose kidney function is greatly reduced, a low-protein diet may be warranted.

My doctor told me I'm losing protein in my urine. Should I eat more protein to replace it?

Taking insulin may be a part of your diabetes regimen, and may be essential to helping to control your diabetes. However, insulin by itself does not protect the kidneys.

Will insulin help protect my kidneys?

Researchers have found that the intensive management of blood sugars may help to slow or prevent the development of kidney failure in Type I and Type II diabetics. A regimen that produces blood sugars as close to normal as possible is best. Some patients require frequent insulin administrations (or even an insulin pump) to accomplish this. Talk to your doctor about whether or not these options are best for you.

What should my blood sugars be to best protect my kidneys?

You should be familiar with a test called the "hemoglobin A1C." This is a blood test that gives a general average of your blood sugars over the last 3 months. It should be kept at less than 7 percent. Your doctor should check your A1C at least twice a year.

I also have high blood pressure. What should my blood pressure be to best protect my kidneys?

High blood pressure is a major factor in the development of kidney disease in diabetics. Over time, high blood pressure damages the blood vessels supplying the kidneys, causing parts of the kidney to die. This process is called nephrosclerosis.

The American Diabetes Association and the Joint National Committee on the Prevention, Detection, Evaluation, and Treatment of High Blood Pressure have each recommended that the blood pressure in a diabetic patient be kept below 130/80. This can be achieved with medications as well as through dietary and lifestyle modifications recommended by your doctor.

Will taking vitamins help?

Vitamin supplementation may be an important part of your medication regimen at certain stages of kidney disease. However, vitamins on their own will not prevent or reverse the development of kidney disease.

All vitamin supplements you take should be recommended by or evaluated by your doctor and/or dietician, as certain substances often found in vitamins (such as potassium, calcium, and excess vitamin C) may be harmful for patients with advanced kidney disease.

My blood sugars are getting lower recently. Does this mean my diabetes is getting better?

Assuming that your diabetes medications have not been changed recently, a more likely explanation for lower blood sugars may have to do with the way your medications are handled by the kidneys. Insulin and certain other diabetes medications are metabolized by the kidneys. When kidney function is decreased, these medications are not metabolized as quickly and therefore remain active in the body for a longer period of time. Thus, as kidney failure progresses, blood sugar control often improves, and you may require a reduction in your insulin or other diabetes medications to avoid dangerously low blood sugars.

Should you notice that your blood sugars are dropping, be sure to inform your physician as soon as possible.

Two kinds of blood pressure medications may help protect the kidneys of diabetic patients who don't necessarily have high blood pressure. These medications are known as angiotensin-converting enzyme (ACE) inhibitors and angiotensin receptor blockers (ARBs). Both types of medications may reduce the amount of protein being lost in the urine and can lead to improved long-term survival of the kidneys.

Why did my doctor put me on high blood pressure medications even though I don't have high blood pressure?

Some evidence exists that beneficial effects may be seen in patients taking both classes of drugs in combination. Your doctor will decide on the best medication regimen for you. Obviously, do not take any medications without the knowledge and advice of your physician.

Dialysis is a therapy that is able to clear the blood of toxic waste products in patients who progress to advanced kidney failure. There are two major types of dialysis: hemodialysis and peritoneal dialysis. In hemodialysis, the patient is connected to a machine at a dialysis center for 3-4 hours, three times a week. The dialysis machine filters the patient's blood and returns it to the patient. In peritoneal dialysis, a permanent catheter is surgically inserted into the patient's abdomen. Dialysis solution is infused 3-4 times per day through the catheter into the belly, and this fluid is able to clean the blood of toxic products before it is removed a few hours later. Peritoneal dialysis can be done by the patient at home.

If I need dialysis, what are my options?

The appropriate method of dialysis for you will be discussed with you by your doctor if it appears you will need dialysis. However, it must be stressed that not all diabetics with kidney disease advance to the need for dialysis, and therefore it is very important that you meet with your doctor frequently to help protect your kidneys in order to possibly avoid dialysis altogether. (See also Chapter 3.)

I've heard that diabetics cannot have peritoneal dialysis. Is this true?

No. Certain peritoneal dialysis solutions contain sugar, and this sugar can be absorbed through the peritoneum into the blood. Thus, diabetics on peritoneal dialysis occasionally develop higher blood sugars. This can often be controlled by a medication adjustment. Also, newer dialysis solutions may use substances other than sugar and may be better for diabetic patients. Peritoneal dialysis remains an important option in kidney replacement among diabetic patients.

Once I am on dialysis, will I still need insulin?

Dialysis does not cure diabetes, and diabetes has other very important effects on organs other than the kidney. Diabetics who have uncontrolled blood sugars are at higher risk for blindness, nerve damage, and cardiovascular disease even once on dialysis. Thus, it is extremely important to continue close monitoring of your diabetes, and to continue the medications your doctor prescribes. You should continue to see your doctors and a dietician on a regular basis. You should also continue to check your blood sugars and take those results to your doctor during your routine visits.

Can I get a transplant? What are the benefits? Can we talk about Kidney Pancreas Transplant?

Yes. Kidney transplantation remains the best option for most diabetic patients with kidney failure. In some patients (particularly Type I diabetics), simultaneous kidney and pancreas transplant may be a viable option. Multiple studies have shown that survival and quality of life are significantly improved in kidney failure patients who undergo a transplant versus remaining on dialysis. In addition, transplant patients no longer need to go to hemodialysis sessions multiple times per week.

Living donor transplantation, if available to you, has the best outcomes, and the transplanted kidney may last the rest of your life. If a donor is available, transplantation can occur even prior to your starting dialysis. In fact, the best transplant outcomes are seen in patients that were transplanted before they needed dialysis. It is advisable to begin speaking with family members and/or friends about their thoughts on kidney donation as soon as possible.

The current waiting list varies for a deceased donor transplant and can be as long as 4-6 years, depending on your blood type. Therefore, patients who require a deceased donor should be placed on the transplant wait list by their nephrologist as soon as possible. Be sure to discuss your transplant options with your physician!

Will my diabetes get worse after a transplant?

Transplant recipients are required to take medications to prevent rejection for the rest of their life. Some of these medications (one of which is prednisone, a steroid), may cause blood sugars to rise. Another frequently used anti-rejection medication, tacrolimus, has been shown to occasionally cause diabetes in previous non-diabetic patients, and may worsen diabetic control in pre-existing diabetic patients. The doses of these medications are reduced by the transplant physicians over time, but still may cause a worsening of your blood sugar control.

You may require insulin to control your blood sugars, even if you never required insulin prior to the transplant. The doses of your diabetic medications will also need to be adjusted, so close follow-up by your doctors will be required after the transplant surgery.

Will the diabetes affect a transplanted kidney? If your diabetes continues to be uncontrolled after the transplant surgery, your transplant kidney may suffer the same fate as your original (native) kidneys. However, as described above, it may take up to ten years for diabetes to begin affecting the transplanted kidney, and after that would likely take many years for kidney function to decrease. However, it remains extremely important to control your diabetes after a transplant, not merely for the sake of the transplanted kidney, but also to avoid other health risks to your eyes, nervous system, and heart.

Cardiovascular Complications

Patients with kidney disease are at higher risk of having cardiovascular disease. It is the most common cause of death and is higher in all age groups in patients with end stage kidney disease. Cardiovascular disease may include coronary heart disease (narrowing of the blood vessels in the heart), cerebrovascular disease (stroke), renal artery stenosis (narrowing of the blood vessel to the kidney), peripheral vascular disease (disease of the blood vessels in the arms and legs), congestive heart failure, and left ventricular hypertrophy (LVH). LVH, enlargement of the heart muscle, is the most common heart problem in patients on dialysis.

What is the significance of cardiovascular disease in patients with kidney disease?

Death due to cardiovascular disease is 20 times more frequent in patients with kidney disease than in the general population. The causes include arrhythmia (irregular heart beat), cardiomyopathy (bad heart muscle function), myocardial infarction (heart attack), cardiac arrest (heart stopping), stroke, atherosclerotic heart disease ("hardening of the arteries"), and pulmonary edema (excess lung fluid).

What are the causes of death due to cardiovascular disease in patients with end stage kidney disease?

The incidence of cardiovascular disease in patients with kidney disease is very high. Of all the causes of cardiovascular disease, cardiac arrest or sudden cardiac death is the most common cause of cardiovascular death in patients on dialysis.

What is the incidence of cardiovascular disease in patients with kidney disease?

The traditional risk factors for cardiovascular disease in people without kidney disease are diabetes, hypertension, a past or current history of cigarette smoking, older age, male gender, a family history of cardiovascular disease, abnormal levels of cholesterol in the blood, obesity, little or no exercise, and high blood levels of homocystein.

What are the traditional risk factors of cardiovascular disease in people without kidney disease?

Are there special risk factors for cardiovascular disease in patients with kidney disease?

The risk factors for cardiovascular disease that are specific to patients with kidney disease include uremia, anemia, high levels of parathyroid hormone in the blood, build up of waste products in the blood such as asymmetric dimethyl arginine or ADMA and advanced glycated end products or AGE, chronic systemic inflammation and cardiovascular instability.

Why are patients with kidney disease at greater risk for cardiovascular disease?

Patients with kidney disease are usually at greater risk for cardiovascular disease because they typically suffer from a number of illnesses that may have either caused their kidneys to fail and/or are connected with premature heart disease, such as diabetes. In addition, most patients with kidney disease may have both traditional and unique risk factors for cardiovascular disease.

What are some of the signs of cardiovascular disease in patients with kidney disease?

Some of the signs for cardiovascular disease include shortness of breath, chest pain, swelling in your legs, sudden weakness or paralysis, severe headaches, sudden onset of blurred vision or visual disturbance, or palpitations especially if you are also light-headed.

What should I know about my cholesterol lab values?

You should know that your cholesterol labs are made up of several parts. The parts are the total cholesterol level, the LDL or low-density lipoprotein cholesterol (sometimes referred to as the 'bad' cholesterol), the HDL or high-density lipoprotein cholesterol (sometimes referred to as the 'good cholesterol') and the triglyceride level. There are guidelines for achieving and maintaining desirable levels of total cholesterol (<200 mg/dl), LDL cholesterol (<100 mg/dl), HDL cholesterol (>40 mg/dl) and triglyceride level (<150 mg/dl). Your doctor will regularly monitor these levels with blood tests and may place you on medications to help manage these levels.

Diabetes is the most common cause of end stage kidney disease, followed by hypertension. Having diabetes, even without kidney disease, increases the risk of cardiovascular disease similar to an individual with a history of heart disease. Having kidney disease with both diabetes and hypertension places you at greater risk of developing a cardiac condition than having either diabetes alone or hypertension alone. As a result, it is important to work with your doctor to make sure that both your diabetes and hypertension are well controlled in order to limit these risks.

How does having either diabetes or hypertension impact my risk for cardiovascular disease?

In addition to all of the benefits already discussed, correction of your anemia will improve your heart function and allow your heart to have greater exercise tolerance. Exercise tolerance may be even better when your blood pressure is also improved. Your doctor will give you recombinant erythropoietin or a similar medication, to help correct your anemia.

How does correcting my anemia impact my risk for cardiovascular disease?

In general, your anemia should be corrected to a hemoglobin level of 11 g/dl to 12 g/dl and a hematocrit of 33% to 36%.

What levels should my anemia be corrected to?

High levels of parathyroid hormone, or hyperparathyroidism, causes excess calcification (calcium deposits) within the walls of the blood vessels in patients receiving dialysis. It may be seen as calcification of the arteries or coronaries of the heart. This may contribute to premature cardiovascular disease and increase the risk of death from heart disease.

How does having high levels of parathyroid hormone impact my cardiovascular risk?

How can I reduce my parathyroid hormone levels? You can reduce your parathyroid hormone to acceptable levels by following instructions from your doctor and nutritionist to limit intake of foods that are high in calcium and phosphate and by taking medicine prescribed by your doctor. In some cases, the parathyroid gland may need to be removed.

Will maintaining my parathyroid hormone levels reduce my cardio-vascular risk? Studies have shown that removal of the parathyroid gland in dialysis patients in whom this was indicated resulted in improved function of the heart muscle.

How can I lower my risks of dying from cardiovascular disease? You can help to lower your cardiovascular risk factors by managing your diet, body weight, exercise, cholesterol level, blood pressure, anemia, and reducing/stopping smoking. In addition to discussion with your physician, and nutritionist, there are several websites which provide useful information to assist in managing those cardiovascular risk factors that are known to be changeable.

Diet:
www.nutrition.gov;
Body weight:
www.nhlbi.nih.gov/subsites/index.htm
(go to Healthy Weight);
Exercise:
www.fitness.gov/aboutpcpfs/aboutpcpfs.html;
Cholesterol:
www.nhlbi.nih.gov.chd;
Blood pressure:
www.nhlbi.nih.gov/hbp;
Hormone replacement:
www.nhlbi.nih.gov/whi/hrtupd/index.htm;
Cigarette smoking:
www.cdc.gov/tobacco/sgr_tobacco_use.htm.

Renal Bone Disease

As the "master chemists" of the body, kidneys play a key role in controlling how the body handles calcium and phosphorus—the minerals that make up bone. The kidneys are also responsible for turning vitamin D into an active hormone. Active vitamin D causes the intestines to absorb calcium and phosphorus. It is also responsible for these minerals being put into bone. As kidney function worsens, active vitamin D levels drop. This causes low blood calcium levels which causes bones to release calcium and phosphorus to try to maintain normal blood levels. Low blood calcium levels cause the parathyroid gland to produce more parathyroid hormone (PTH).

Why does kidney disease cause bone disease?

In advanced kidney disease, especially in people on dialysis, the kidneys cannot get rid of phosphorus. High blood phosphorus levels cause PTH levels to further increase. High PTH causes the bone to release more calcium and phosphorus to keep blood calcium levels normal. These minerals come out of the bone and weaken the skeleton. Children grow poorly. Both adults and children will have more bone deformities and fractures.

Vitamin D is produced in the skin when you are in the sunshine. It can also be absorbed through the intestines from certain foods. The kidney is responsible for changing the vitamin D, made in the skin and absorbed from food into an active hormone. This hormone increases the amount of calcium absorbed from the diet, and puts the calcium into bone. In kidney disease, vitamin D can no longer be changed to an active form, so active vitamin D is given as a medicine, either orally or intravenously. Three active vitamin D medications that may be prescribed for you are:

How does the kidney regulate vitamin D?

1) Rocaltrol® (calcitriol)

2) Zemplar® (paricalcitol)

3) Hectoral® (doxercalciferol).

When does renal bone disease start and how is it monitored?

The kidneys' ability to make vitamin D goes down when about half of normal kidney function is gone. This can happen a long time before the kidneys completely stop working. Therefore calcium, phosphorus, and PTH levels in the blood may be checked often in people a long time before they require dialysis.

Does diet affect bone disease?

Extra phosphorus in the blood worsens bone disease. Phosphorus is found in a variety of foods including dairy products, meat, eggs, and most sodas. While it is important for people with kidney disease to eat enough protein to stay healthy, phosphorus comes along with protein. Eating too much protein increases blood phosphorus levels. It is important to discuss your diet with a renal dietician in order to eat healthy foods while avoiding extra phosphorus.

Does dialysis control phosphorus levels?

Dialysis does remove some phosphorus from the blood. However, a typical hemodialysis or peritoneal dialysis treatment regimen will remove, on average, less than half the phosphorus that a person on a healthy diet should eat.

What are phosphate binders?

Healthy kidneys regulate the amount of phosphorus in the blood and get rid of extra phosphorus in the urine. In people with advanced kidney disease and on dialysis, phosphorus builds up in the blood. Therefore most people who are on dialysis need medicine to keep blood phosphorus levels normal. These medications are called "phosphate binders." They combine with the phosphorus in foods and prevent the phosphorous from going into the blood. Commonly used phosphate binders are:

1) Tums® or OsCal® (calcium carbonate), Phoslo® (calcium acetate)

2) Renagel® (sevelamer hydrochloride)
3) Alu-Caps® (aluminum) or Fosrenol® (lanthanum carbonate)

How does vitamin D work to control PTH?

PTH levels are controlled by maintaining normal blood phosphorus levels (by limiting the amount of phosphorus eaten and by taking phosphate binders) and by treatment with vitamin D. Vitamin D is often given as an intravenous medication during hemodialysis. It may also be given orally for people who are treated with peritoneal dialysis or for those who do not yet need dialysis. Vitamin D causes the intestines to absorb calcium, preventing both low blood calcium levels and excess PTH secretion. At the same time, vitamin D lowers PTH by preventing it from being made in the parathyroid glands.

What other ways are PTH levels controlled?

Sensipar®, also called cinacalcet, is often useful in lowering PTH levels when vitamin D and phosphorus control are not working. Sensipar tricks the parathyroid glands into thinking that more calcium is in the blood than is actually there, so the glands produce less PTH. Sometimes, however, despite large doses of vitamin D, good control of blood phosphorus levels, and the use of Sensipar®, the parathyroid glands still produce too much PTH. If this occurs, some people require surgery to remove the parathyroid glands.

Is it possible to suppress PTH too much?

Use of too much vitamin D may cause PTH levels to drop to low levels which may make the bones very brittle. This is called adynamic bone disease. It is a condition, in which bones fracture much more easily than healthy bones. Many people with kidney disease from diabetes have low PTH levels and adynamic bone disease, even without taking any vitamin D.

Do medications for bone disease have side effects?

As with most medications, there are side effects to the medicines used to treat renal bone disease. Use of large amounts of Tums®, Oscal®, or Phoslo® (calcium carbonate or calcium acetate) may cause too much calcium to be absorbed into the body. The extra calcium will be deposited in blood vessels and other tissues, which may cause heart disease (see cardiovascular chapter). Large amounts of vitamin D may also cause excess absorption of calcium and phosphorus which also contributes to cardiovascular disease. These side effects are lessened by using types of vitamin D that decrease the amount of calcium and phosphorus absorbed, and by using phosphate binders that don't contain calcium.

Alu-Caps® (aluminum hydroxide) is a metal containing phosphate binder that is partly absorbed if used in high doses over a long period of time. Aluminum is then deposited in bone and causes a form of bone disease. Aluminum can also cause problems with neurologic (brain) function.

Fosrenol® (lanthanum carbonate) is a newer medication which also contains a metal, some of which may be absorbed and deposited in the body. Since it is a new medication, studies are being done to determine if it causes any long-term problems.

Sensipar® (cinacalcet) may cause blood calcium and phosphorus levels to drop. It may also cause some stomach irritation.

Advance Directives

Introduction

Today, medical advances have made it possible for many diseases to be treated successfully, adding to life expectancy and quality of life. However, life-saving advances sometimes mean watching someone you love being kept alive when you are not sure what his or her choice would have been about the treatment being given. Often, doctors and families are asked to make difficult treatment decisions. In some cases, the courts have been called on to make these decisions.

Many decisions can be made by patients and their families before a medical crisis occurs. Patients with kidney disease might consider preparing a legal document to guide loved ones, doctors and other health care professionals in providing treatment in a time of crisis.

The Patient Self-Determination Act, in effect since 1991, gives adults with the capacity to make medical decisions for themselves the right to make decisions today about health care treatment they would want to receive in the future if they could not communicate what they want at that time. This law requires that hospitals, nursing homes and other health agencies give all patients information about their right to have a legal document called an advance directive. Dialysis units are not legally required to give you this information, but the National Kidney Foundation and many dialysis units believe dialysis patients should know about the right to make an advance directive.

What is an Advance Directive?

An advance directive is a legal paper that tells doctors and health care providers how you want them to carry out medical decisions you have made for future crisis care, even if you cannot communicate these decisions for yourself. If you have an advance directive in your medical records, your doctor and other health care providers can take care of you based on your wishes as stated in the advance directive.

There are two basic kinds of advance directives:

- A living will, the more common type, tells your doctor or health care provider in writing what type of medical care you want or do not want if you should become unable to make these decisions for yourself.
- A durable power of attorney for health care decisions, or a health care proxy allows you to name someone, such as a husband, wife, daughter, son or close friend, to act on your behalf if you are unable to make medical decisions for yourself. It is important to ask this person if he or she is willing to act as your "agent" and to talk about what treatments you would want and those you would not want, as well as your short- and long-term goals and values.

Your state's laws may allow you to have both a living will and a durable power of attorney or to combine them in a single form. You may want to speak to a lawyer or contact your state or local bar association about your state's laws concerning advance directives.

Could my family or friend just decide for me without an advance directive?

Laws are strict about this. Hospitals and other health care providers usually will not let a friend decide unless he or she is named in an advance directive. Without an advance directive, your family may have to go to court to have treatment stopped.

With an advance directive, it may be possible to accept all treatments recommended by the health care provider, accept some treatments and refuse others, or refuse all recommended treatments.

In your advance directive, you can choose to receive pain medicines for comfort even if you refuse other treatments. You may be able to accept or refuse other treatments, such as:

- Cardiopulmonary resuscitation (CPR) to restore breathing and blood circulation. (This includes heart massage, drugs, electric shocks and artificial breathing machines.)
- Tube feedings, including giving food and/or water through a tube into a vein or into the stomach.
- Artificial respiration (ventilator or respirator), which is a machine that breathes for a person through a tube in the throat.
- Antibiotics to fight infection.
- Dialysis for kidney failure, either hemodialysis or peritoneal dialysis.
- Surgery such as heart bypass, gall bladder, etc.
- Blood transfusions or blood products; you may also decide whether you would only want blood from your family members or friends.

Some states may limit your ability to delegate to someone else the authority to refuse one or more types of treatment, for example, providing artificial nutrition or water. Some states may require that treatment be continued once it is accepted by your surrogate. It is important to speak with a lawyer or social worker, or get a copy of your state's advance directive forms so you will understand your state's specific laws.

Advance Directives and Dialysis

Can an advance directive state the conditions under which dialysis could be stopped?

Yes. An advance directive allows you to tell your doctor, family and loved ones the specific conditions that you feel would limit the quality of life you want for yourself. You may choose to stop dialysis if you have brain damage (caused by a stroke, Alzheimer's disease, etc.), if you cannot move independently (due to a stroke, paralysis, etc.) or if you have to depend totally on others. These are a few of the specific conditions that you can state in an advance directive. In contrast, you may state that you want to live under any condition.

If a patient chooses to stop dialysis, how would he or she die?

Deaths from kidney failure do not have to be unpleasant. If kidney failure is allowed to take its natural course, there will be a build-up of toxic wastes from food and the breakdown of body tissues. Fluid will build up in the tissues, which may cause the patient to become short of breath. The doctor may prescribe diuretics or a type of dialysis (ultrafiltration) that only removes fluid, to make breathing easier. Pain medicines may be prescribed if there appears to be any discomfort. The length of time a dialysis patient can live without treatment varies. If a patient chooses to stop dialysis, hospice services (which may include nursing care, social work and chaplain services) may be available to help. Medicare and insurance can help pay for these services. If you have any questions about stopping dialysis, speak with your health care team.

Other Important Points

- You are not required by law to have an advance directive.
- You do not need to see a lawyer to make an advance directive; however, you may want to speak to a lawyer or social worker to fully understand your state's laws.
- You can get advance directive forms from your state or local bar association, most senior citizen centers,

some health care providers, state health department web sites or www.partnershipforcaring.org

- You can list the treatments you would want or not want without using a form, but a court or medical provider may not accept them.
- State laws may require that advance directives be witnessed or notarized. Banks and other business have notaries who can do this.
- You should speak to your doctor before making an advance directive. He or she can explain treatment options and tell you whether he or she would object to carrying out your choices.
- Be sure to tell the necessary people about your advance directive. The only way your family, friends, doctor or health care providers will know you have one is if you tell them. It can be made a part of your medical record.
- If you change your advance directive, you need to tell everyone you have given copies to and give them the new one. If you cancel it, you need to get back all of the copies.
- If you are religious, you may wish to speak with your family and your religious advisor to understand your religion's views in regard to advance directives.
- An advance directive goes into effect only if and when you are not able to communicate and make your own health care decisions.
- Having an advance directive does not affect the quality of your care.
- Having an advance directive does not affect life or health insurance.
- Your wishes for donating organs or tissues can be stated in your advance directive. It is also important to tell your family and friends about your wishes so they will carry them out.

Discussion Topics Talking about the following questions with a family member or a close friend may help you understand how you feel about these life and death issues.

- What is the minimum quality of life acceptable to you?
- What are your attitudes toward death?
- How important are being independent and making your own decisions to you?
- Do you have any health problems now? How would you describe them?
- Would your religious beliefs affect your attitude toward life-sustaining treatments? If so, which ones?
- If you were terminally ill with no hope of recovery, which life-sustaining treatments would you want to continue?
- If you have severe and permanent brain damage, would you want any life-sustaining treatments would you want to continue? If so, which ones?
- If you were in a permanent coma, would you want any life-sustaining treatments to continue? If so, which ones?
- Do you feel your family and friends would support you in your decisions about future medical care?
- Who would you want to speak for you and state your decisions if you were unable to express them yourself? Would this person be agreeable to doing this?
- Would you want to donate any organs or tissues (heart, kidneys, liver, eyes, bone) to someone else at the time of your death? Specify what organs or tissues, if any, you would want to donate.

Talk to members of your health care team or any health care provider who must give you information about advance directives. Talk with your lawyer, your local bar association or to the Legal Aid Society in your community. Also, see the list of resources below.

Where can I get more information?

Partnership for Caring
1620 Eye Street NW, Suite 202
Washington, DC 20006
Phone: (800) 989-WILL or (202) 296-8071
Internet: www.partnershipforcaring.org

Other Resources

American Bar Association
Commission on Legal Problems of the Elderly
740 15th Street, NW
Washington, DC 20005-1022
(202) 662-8690
E-mail: abaelderly@abanet.org
Internet: www.abanet.org/elderly
Video In Your Hands: *The Tools for Preserving Personal Autonomy* may be rented or purchased. Booklets on advance directives are also available for purchase.

In order to be prepared for a possible medical crisis, you may want to make sure the following items are in order:

Checklist of Things to Consider

- Your will.
- Signed advance directive (living will, durable health care power of attorney or health care proxy) complying with your state law.
- A durable power of attorney, complying with your state law, naming someone to act on your behalf on all matters other than medical (legal, financial, banking and business matters). Your power of attorney must be a "durable" one in order for it to stay in effect even if you become unable to make your own decisions or if you die.
- An inventory, including location of your bank,

brokerage and other financial accounts, stock and bond holdings, real estate and business records, medical and other insurance policies, pension plans and other legal papers.

- Names, addresses and telephone numbers of your attorney, accountant, family members and other loved ones, friends and business associates who should be notified of your death or who may have information that will be helpful in dealing with estate affairs.

- A statement about your preference for funeral/memorial services, burial or cremation instructions and decisions about organ and tissue donation.

- Written, videotaped or audiotaped message to family members and other loved ones, business associates and friends.

- All health information in this chapter has been approved for medical accuracy by the Scientific Advisory Board of the National Kidney Foundation. This information was current as of the date of publication.

This chapter is based on the Advance Directives pamphlet of the National Kidney Foundation and is included here with their permission.

For a more comprehensive discussion of advance directives please see Appendix G.

Acquired immune deficiency syndrome (AIDS): The multiplicity of implications that may follow a viral infection that attacks the body's immune system, making the patient unable to fight off other serious infections.

Acute kidney failure: A condition in which the kidneys suddenly stop working. In most cases, kidneys can recover from almost complete loss of function.

Acute tubular necrosis (ATN): A severe form of acute renal failure that develops in people with severe illness like infections or with low blood pressure.

Acute: Acute often means urgent. An acute disease happens suddenly. It lasts a short time. Acute is the opposite of chronic, or long lasting.

ADMA: Refers to asymmetric dimethyl arginine which is a substance produced in cells that make up blood vessels. It is strongly associated with insulin resistance and increases with reducing kidney function. It is associated with high cardiovascular risk in the general population, patients with kidney disease and patients with complete kidney failure.

Advance directive: A statement made by an individual to guide his or her treatment or to indicate whom the individual would like to make health care decisions for him or her should he or she become unable to make decisions. If appropriately written and witnessed the advance directive is a legal document.

Agent, agent-in fact, attorney-in-fact: Interchangeable terms for the individual (often called a proxy or surrogate) appointed in an advance directive by the principal to make healthcare decisions for the principal after the principal has become incapable of making healthcare decisions.

Agent, Agent-in-fact, Attorney-in-fact: These three terms are interchangeable. They name the person officially appointed or designated in writing by an individual to act on his or her behalf should he or she become incapable of making health care decisions.

AGEs: Are generated in response to chronic excess circulating glucose in the blood in which glucose molecules are added to proteins and lipid which then accumulate in blood vessels, kidneys and tissues in patients with diabetes. In patients, high levels of AGEs correlate with increased levels of hemoglobin A1C, which is measure of the level of control of diabetes, increased levels of albumin in the urine, the duration of diabetes and high levels of fasting plasma glucose.

Albumin: The most common protein found in the blood.

Albuminuria: More than normal amounts of protein called albumin in the urine.

Allergic: Being unusually sensitive to a particular substance (for example, a drug, grass or food).

Allograft: An organ or tissue transplant between two humans.

Aluminum intoxication: The build up of aluminum in the body, which can cause a disorder called dialysis dementia or aluminum bone disease.

Amyloidosis: A condition in which a protein-like material builds up in one or more organs. This material cannot be broken down and interferes with the normal function of that organ.

Analgesic-associated kidney disease: The loss of kidney function that results from long-term use of analgesic medications.

Analgesics: Medications that relieve pain and, in some cases, reduce fever.

Anemia: The condition of having too few red blood cells. Healthy red blood cells carry oxygen throughout the body. If the blood is low on red blood cells, the body does not get enough oxygen.

Anemic: Having anemia or less than the normal number of red blood cells in the blood.

Angina: Chest pain caused by a reduced blood supply to the heart muscle.

Antacid: Medications that block or neutralize stomach acid, some of which are also used as phosphate binders.

Antibiotics: Medications that either stop the growth of bacteria or kill bacteria.

Antibody: A body substance that fights off disease and foreign substances or reacts against body tissue.

Anticoagulants: A type of medication that prevents blood from clotting.

Antidiuretic hormone: A natural body chemical that slows down the urine flow.

Anuria: A condition in which the person stops making urine.

Arrhythmia: Refers to abnormal heart rhythm.

Arteriovenous fistula (AV fistula): The surgical connection of an artery directly to a vein, usually in the forearm, created in patients who will need hemodialysis. The AV fistula causes the vein to grow thicker, allowing the repeated needle insertions required for hemodialysis.

Artery: Vessel carrying blood away from the heart.

Artificial kidney machine: Refers to a hemodialysis machine though which a patient's blood is circulated in order to maintain the chemical and fluid balance of the body.

Artificial kidney: Refers to a dialyzer.

Atherosclerotic heart disease: Refers to heart disease that occurs as a result of accumulation of lipids in the coronary arteries.

Autoimmune disease: Any disorder in which the body is attacked by its own immune system.

Bacteria: Refers to germs.

Best interests: A basis of healthcare decision-making that considers what would be best for the individual. When this judgment is made by a surrogate or proxy or agent for an individual who has lost decision making capacity, it should be made from the perspective of the individual not the perspective of the person making the decision. Normally it would be made with the advice or consultation of the patient's physician. This basis for decision making should be undertaken only if the principal has not made explicit statements as to what he or she would wish under the circumstances and if the principal's relevant values and goals are not known and thus do not allow for substituted judgment.

Biopsy: A procedure in which a tiny piece of a body part, such as the kidney or bladder, is removed for examination under a microscope.

Biotechnology: Using biology to solve problems relating to humans and disease; see also recombinant DNA technology.

Bladder: The balloon-shaped organ inside the pelvis that holds urine.

Blood flow rate: The rate at which blood flows through the dialyzer.

Blood leaks: Refers to a leak in the membrane of the dialyzer.

Blood pressure: Pressure of the blood flowing through the blood vessels.

Blood urea nitrogen (BUN): A waste product in the blood that comes from the breakdown of food protein. The kidneys filter blood to remove urea.

Blood vessel: Refers to either an artery or a vein.

Bone Marrow: The soft material filling the cavities of the bones where blood cells are produced.

Cadaver donor: See deceased donor.

Calcitonin: A hormone secreted by the thyroid gland that protects against the loss of minerals in the bones and counter-balances the effects of parathyroid and Vitamin D.

Calcium: A mineral that the body needs for strong bones and teeth.

Capillary dialyzer: A type of dialyzer consisting of thousands of tiny plastic tubes through which a patient's blood flows.

Cardiac arrest: When the heart stops beating.

Cardiomyopathy: Refers to an abnormality of the heart muscle.

Cardiopulmonary resuscitation (CPR): A coordinated the set of treatments for the purpose of reestablishing cardiac (heart) and pulmonary (lung) function when either the heart stops beating or the lungs stop breathing or both. The treatments consist of breathing for the patient (usually via a mask or a tube in the windpipe) and of manually compressing the chest to "massage" the heart in order to pump blood throughout the body. Oxygen and medications are usually given, and if the electrical activity of the heart is deranged (ventricular fibrillation), electric shock may be delivered to the heart by electrodes applied to the chest wall in an effort to restore a normal heart rhythm and beat. The purpose, of course, is to prevent death and, by prompt initiation of CPR, to prevent brain damage.

Catheter: A plastic or rubber tube through which fluids enter or leave the body.

Cell: A microscopic entity capable of performing all of the basic functions of life (moving, reproduction, etc.)

Cerebrovascular disease: Refers to atherosclerotic disease of the cerebral or brain arteries that causes strokes and transient ischemic attacks.

CHD or coronary heart disease: Refers to atherosclerotic disease of the coronary arteries that causes myocardial ischemia

Chloramines: A type of disinfectant used in some tap water that must be removed from water used in artificial kidney machines.

Chronic kidney disease: A slow and progressive loss of kidney function over several years, often resulting in severe loss of kidney function, which will eventually require dialysis or transplantation.

Chronic: Lasting a long time. Chronic diseases develop slowly.

Clear and convincing (an evidentiary standard): A standard in law requiring evidence of very high quality, and as quoted in the California Supreme Court ruling in the case of Robert Wendland, "a finding of high probability based on evidence... so clear as to leave no substantial doubt [and] sufficiently strong to command the unhesitating assent of every reasonable mind."

Combined or comprehensive advance directive: An advance directive consisting of both a proxy directive and a treatment directive.

Competence (competency): The legal term for decision-making capacity, which requires 1) understanding of one's diagnosis; 2) ability to analyze risks and benefits of possible treatments as well as to understand the consequences of no treatment; and 3) the ability to make and state a choice or decision.

Conservator: A court-appointed guardian (a person or an agency) to manage the affairs or property of an incompetent person.

Continuous Ambulatory Peritoneal Dialysis (CAPD): A form of peritoneal dialysis in which the dialysate is in the peritoneum 24 hours a day, seven days a week, where the patient infuses solution by hand.

Continuous Cycling Peritoneal Dialysis (CCPD): A form of peritoneal dialysis that uses a machine and can be done at home.

Creatinine clearance: A test that measures how efficiently the kidneys remove creatinine and other wastes from the blood.

Creatinine: A waste product from meat protein in the diet and is a by-product of normal muscle metabolism.

CVD or cardiovascular disease: Refers to coronary heart disease, cerebrovascular disease, renal artery stenosis, peripheral vascular disease, congestive heart failure, or left ventricular hypertrophy.

Cycler: The dialysis machine used in continuous cycling peritoneal dialysis (CCPD).

Cyst: An abnormal sac containing gas, fluid, or a semisolid material.

Deceased donor: Term used for the nonliving, unrelated person whose kidney is used as a transplant organ for another person.

Decisional incapacity: The lack of decision-making capacity.

Decision-making capacity (decisional capacity): The ability to make decisions for oneself which in common language is called "competence." It requires an understanding of one's situation (illness or diagnosis and prognosis); the expected consequences of the illness; the nature, probable outcome, and possible risks of proposed and alternative treatments and of no treatment; the ability to reason about the alternatives weighing their benefits and burdens; and to make or state a choice or decision. One is presumed to have decision-making capacity until and unless demonstrated to the contrary. Unlike "competence" which requires a determination in court, decision-making capacity can be determined by a physician.

Dextrose: A sugar solution found in peritoneal dialysate that may also be added to the dialysate in hemodialysis.

Diabetes insipidus: A condition characterized by frequent and heavy urination, excessive thirst, and an overall feeling of weakness. In diabetes insipidus, blood sugar levels are normal.

Diabetes mellitus: A condition characterized by high blood sugar resulting from the body's inability to use sugar (glucose) efficiently. In type 1 diabetes, the pancreas is not able to make enough insulin; in type 2 diabetes, the body is resistant to the effects of available insulin.

Diabetic nephropathy: Kidney failure resulting from diabetes when damaged blood vessels make the kidneys unable to filter the blood properly.

Dialysate: Solution used in dialysis to remove excess fluids and waste products from the blood.

Dialysis dementia: A neurological disorder that may be caused by aluminum intoxication or high levels of aluminum in the body.

Dialysis: The process of artificially maintaining the chemical balance and cleaning wastes from the blood.

Dialyzer: That part of the hemodialysis system that contains the artificial membrane through which blood passes during hemodialysis.

Diffusion: The method used during dialysis to remove waste products from the blood and to balance chemicals in the blood.

DNA: The material of cells that carries the genetic code.

Do Not Resuscitate (DNR) order: See DNAR.

Do-not-attempt resuscitation order (DNAR): An order, written by a physician, to alert healthcare professionals to honor a decision not to attempt cardiopulmonary resuscitation should a cardiac (heart) and/or pulmonary (lung) arrest occur. The request for such an order may be made by a patient or, especially if the patient is decisionally incapacitated, by the patient's family. The order may also be based upon the physician's judgment that cardiopulmonary resuscitation is extremely unlikely to be effective or that it would not be in the patient's best interest. Even then it is generally agreed that the patient or the patient's surrogate should be consulted, and ideally should consent. A minority opinion allows for an independent decision by the physician, preferably with consultant agreement.

Dose: The amount of a drug or therapy to be given at one time.

Dry weight: The weight at which the body's blood pressure is normal and no swelling is present (all excess fluid is removed).

Durable power-of-attorney for healthcare (DPAHC): A written document that appoints another individual (or successor individuals) as proxy to make healthcare decisions on behalf of the principal, usually only after the principal loses the ability to make decisions for him or herself. This delegated power is durable not only in continuing despite loss of decisional capacity by the principal, but also in remaining valid indefinitely (or at least for a number of years) and it may also be valid in allowing post-mortem decisions such as autopsy, disposition of organs, burial or cremation, and funeral or memorial service.

Dwell time: In peritoneal dialysis, the amount of time a bag of dialysate remains in the patient's abdominal cavity during an exchange.

Edema: Swelling caused by too much fluid in the body.

Electrocardiogram (EKG): A tracing of the electrical rhythm of the heart, which is made by an instrument called an electrocardiograph.

Electrolytes: Chemicals in the body fluids that result from the breakdown of salts, including sodium, potassium, magnesium, and chloride.

End-stage renal disease (ESRD): ESRD has the same meaning as the term chronic kidney disease, stage 5, or that stage of kidney damage that requires dialysis or kidney transplantation.

Erythropoietin: A hormone made by the kidneys that helps the bone marrow make red blood cells.

Ethical will: A statement or document (usually personal and informal rather than legal) of an individual who may be terminally-ill and who wishes to leave a personal or spiritual legacy of values. It is a personal statement to one's children or descendents so that one's values will live on.

Euthanasia: Literally, "good death." When the word is used alone it is generally understood to mean active euthanasia which is the putting to death of an individual by another to end the suffering of the individual (often called "mercy killing"). Passive euthanasia (often called "allowing to die") is the omission of life-sustaining treatment to allow an end to suffering which cannot be relieved without anesthesia or death.

Evidentiary standards: Standards for the adequacy of evidence sufficient for a legal decision. Typically a criminal case requires an evidentiary standard of "beyond a reasonable doubt" whereas civil cases require only "the preponderance of the evidence" which is more than 50% likely.

Exchange: A cycle in peritoneal dialysis in which the patient fills the abdominal cavity with dialysate, carries it for a specified dwell time, and then empties the dialysate from the abdomen in preparation for a fresh bag of dialysate.

Expressed wishes: Health care preferences stated clearly by an individual as those he or she would or would not want under specific circumstances.

Fistula: see arteriovenous fistula.

Fluid overload: Refers to a condition in which excess sodium and fluid build up in the body between dialysis treatments.

Folic acid: A substance necessary for red blood cell production.

Full-care facility: An outpatient dialysis center, which may or may not be a hospital.

Gene: A unit of DNA that carries the special genetic code necessary to determine an attribute of a cell or organism.

Genetic code: The information of cells that tell cells what functions they will perform, how they grow, and what they will produce. Altogether, the genetic code determines what characteristics an organism will have.

Glomerular filtration rate: Also known as GFR, this is a number that indicates at what rate the kidneys are filtering the blood.

Glomeruli: plural of glomerulus.

Glomerulonephritis: Inflammation of the glomeruli.

Glomerulosclerosis: Scarring of the glomeruli.

Glomerulus: A tiny set of looping blood vessels in the nephron where blood is filtered in the kidney.

Graft: An internal access device using synthetic material to surgically connect an artery to a vein.

Gram: A unit of weight in the metric system.

Hematocrit: A measure of the amount of red blood cells in the body.

Hematuria: Blood in the urine.

Hemodialysis: The use of a machine to clean wastes from the blood after the kidneys have failed. The blood travels through tubes to a dialyzer, which removes wastes and extra fluid. The cleaned blood then flows through another set of tubes back into the body.

Hemoglobin: The oxygen-carrying pigment of red blood cells; what makes red blood cells red.

Heparin: A substance given to prevent blood from clotting.

Hepatitis A (infectious hepatitis): Can be contracted through close contact with an infected individual. Generally short-lived, and generally results in complete recovery.

Hepatitis B (serum hepatitis): A type of hepatitis transmitted through blood, intimate contact with an infected individual, IV drug abuse and also from an infected mother to the baby. Many people develop chronic hepatitis from hepatitis B, which can cause liver damage, and even liver cancer. Vaccination against hepatitis B is available and recommended for patients with kidney disease.

Hepatitis B antigen test: A test that determines the presence of an antigen associated with a type of hepatitis (serum hepatitis).

Hepatitis C: A form of chronic hepatitis, usually transmitted through blood transfusions or contaminated needles.

Hepatitis: A viral infection of the liver.

Hormone: A natural chemical produced in one part of the body and released into the blood to trigger or regulate particular functions of the body.

Hospice: A program (often a team of healthcare professionals caring for patients in their own home) or an institution that provides palliative care for terminally ill patients. The emphasis is on maintaining comfort and quality-of-life when cure is no longer possible. Attention is paid to emotional, social, and spiritual needs as well as medical. The team typically includes a physician, nurse, social worker, physiotherapist, occupational therapist, pharmacist, chaplain, and sometimes a speech therapist, and music therapist.

Hypercalciuria: Abnormally large amounts of calcium in the urine.

Hyperkalemia: A condition in which high levels of potassium build up in the blood.

Hypertension: High blood pressure, which can be caused either by too much fluid in the blood vessels or by narrowing of the blood vessels.

Hypotension: Abnormally low blood pressure.

Immune system: The body's system for protecting itself from viruses and bacteria or any "foreign" substances.

Immunosuppressant: A drug given to suppress the natural responses of the body's immune system. Immunosuppressants are given to transplanted patients to prevent organ rejection and to patients with autoimmune diseases.

Incompetence (incompetency): In the narrow or legal sense, a lack of decision making capacity as judged by a court of law, or not yet having reached the age of majority that legally entitles individuals to make decisions for themselves. In common language or the broad sense, the lack of decisional capacity need not be a determination of a court.

Informed consent (or refusal): The right to make healthcare decisions for oneself (and to be provided the information necessary to do so in) based on the legal right of self-determination and the ethical principle of autonomy.

Insulin: The hormone produced in the pancreas and used by the tissues to get energy from blood sugar.

Intermittent peritoneal dialysis (IPD): A form of peritoneal dialysis that requires a machine to perform the exchanges and is usually done in a hospital or clinic.

Interstitial nephritis: Inflammation of the kidney cells that are not part of the fluid-collecting units.

Iron: A metallic element found in hemoglobin.

Kidney donor: The person from whom a healthy kidney is taken to be transplanted into another person.

Kidney stone: A stone that develops from crystals that form in urine and build up on the inner surfaces of the kidney, in the renal pelvis or in the ureters.

Kidney transplantation: The removal of a kidney from either a living donor or deceased individual and surgically placed into the person with kidney failure.

Kidneys: The two bean-shaped organs that filter wastes from the blood. The kidneys are located near the middle of the back. They create urine, which is delivered to the bladder through tubes called ureters.

Kt/V: A measurement of dialysis dose. The measurement takes into account the efficiency of the dialyzer, the treatment of time and total volume of urea in the body.

Lipid profile: Refers to the plasma levels of total cholesterol, low-density lipoprotein cholesterol, high-density lipoprotein cholesterol and triglycerides.

Living will: An advance directive of the treatment directive type, but usually limiting treatment that one would wish. It is a written statement made by one who is competent regarding his or her preference for treatment or treatment limitation should specific circumstances develop and should the individual at that time be incapable of making health care decisions for him- or herself.

Lupus: An autoimmune disease also called systemic lupus erythematosus which often causes kidney damage.

MediCaid: A federal-state supported program to pay for healthcare for needy and low-income residents.

MediCal: MediCaid in California.

Medicare: Government-provided medical insurance under the Social Security Act.

Membrane: A thin sheet or layer of tissue that lines a cavity or separates two parts of the body. A membrane can act as a filter, allowing some particles to pass from one part of the body to another while keeping others where they are.

Microalbuminuria: The loss of tiny amounts of albumin in the urine. This is the initial phase of diabetic kidney disease.

Modalities: Refers to different forms of treatment.

Myocardial infarction: Refers to death of the heart muscle.

Natural death act: Legislation allowing one to direct his or her physician to withhold or withdraw life-sustaining treatment (and thereby allow a natural death) in the event of terminal illness (sometimes with the additional requirement of disability or infirmity) or permanent unconsciousness. The California act has been superseded by the Healthcare Decisions Law of 2000 which provides for healthcare decision making for patients lacking capacity and for advance directives.

Nephrectomy: Surgical removal of a kidney.

Nephrogenic diabetes insipidus: Constant thirst and frequent urination because the kidney tubules cannot respond to antidiuretic hormone.

Nephrologist: Refers to a physician who is an internist or pediatrician primarily concerned with the medical treatment of patients with kidney disease or kidney failure.

Nephrology: Scientific study of the kidney.

Nephron: A tiny part of the kidneys. Each kidney is made up of about 1 million nephrons, which are the working units of the kidneys, removing wastes and extra fluids from the blood.

Nephrosclerosis: Scarring and shrinkage of the filtering portions of the kidney. This process is often seen in patients with hypertension.

Nephrotic syndrome: A collection of symptoms that include lots of protein in the urine, low blood proteins, and body swelling.

Neuropathy: Refers to any disease of the nerves that may cause nerve injury and a change in feeling in the feet, legs or hands.

Palliative care: The non-curative treatment of illness with an emphasis on the relief of symptoms such as pain, shortness of breath, nausea, vomiting, diarrhea, loss of appetite, itching, etc. As with hospice, there is an emphasis on comfort (and if patients are terminally-ill, on quality rather than extent of life) with attention to emotional, social, and spiritual as well as medical needs.

Parathyroid gland: One of several small glands located in the neck that releases a hormone that regulates the calcium and phosphorus level in the blood.

Patient self-determination act (PSDA): A federal law enacted in 1990 requiring hospitals, long-term care facilities, hospice programs, home health agencies, and prepaid health plans (HMO's) to provide patients with information about their rights, under state law, to accept or refuse treatment and to formulate advance directives.

Pelvis: The bowl-shaped bone that supports the spine and holds up the digestive, urinary, and reproductive organs. The legs connect to the body at the pelvis.

Peripheral vascular disease: Refers to atherosclerotic disease of arteries that causes ischemia of the extremities.

Peritoneal dialysis (PD): Cleaning the blood by using the lining of the belly (abdomen) as a filter. A cleansing solution, called dialysate, is drained from a bag into the belly. Fluids and wastes flow through the lining of the belly and remain "trapped" in the dialysate. The dialysate is then drained from the belly, removing the extra fluids and wastes from the body.

Peritoneum: The abdominal cavity.

Peritonitis: Refers to an infection inside the abdominal cavity and may be a complication of peritoneal dialysis.

Phosphate binders: Medication given to prevent the phosphorus in food from being absorbed into the body.

Phosphorus: An important element of the body which, when combined with calcium, helps form bones. Excess levels of phosphorus, however, can rob the bones of much needed calcium.

Physician-assisted suicide: Euthanasia in which the physician prescribes, but the patient takes, a lethal dose of medication to end suffering. In the United States the practice is legal only in the state of Oregon which allows it only in competent, terminally ill patients who voluntarily, informedly, and persistently request it and who personally take the medication.

Polycystic kidney disease (PKD): An inherited disorder characterized by many grape-like clusters of fluid-filled cysts that make both kidneys larger over time. These cysts take over and destroy working kidney tissue.

Potassium: A mineral needed by the body for normal heart and muscle function. Excess potassium in the body, or hyperkalemia, may be harmful.

Proteinuria: The presence of protein in the urine, indicating that the kidneys are not working properly.

Proxy directive: Names the individual or successor individuals who are able to make health care decisions for a patient should he or she become unable to state decisions.

Proxy: A surrogate decision-maker, i.e., an individual authorized or appointed to act for another. Legally an individual designated in an advance directive to make decisions for an individual, usually beginning only when that individual has become decisionally incapacitated. If there is no advance directive, the proxy may be appointed by a court or simply recognized as the legally valid surrogate decision-maker as determined by statute or by common-law (precedent of court decisions in prior cases).

Public guardian: A legally appointed caretaker of an individual who is a minor or who is incapable of administering his or her own affairs.

Pulmonary edema: Refers to accumulation of excessive amount of fluid in the lungs.

Pyelonephritis: An infection of the kidney(s), usually caused by a germ that has traveled up through the urethra, bladder and ureter from outside the body.

Recombinant DNA technology: The process of placing different genes into a cell to change the genetic make-up of the cell; it will alter the cell so that the cell will do things it would not do otherwise.

Recombinant human erythropoietin: A hormone made through biotechnology that is very similar to the natural hormone (erythropoietin), which stimulates the production of red blood cells in the bone marrow.

Red blood cells: The oxygen-carrying cells of the bloodstream.

Rejection: The body's means of destroying the presence of a foreign substance or tissue from an outside source.

Renal agenesis: The absence or severe malformation of one or both kidneys.

Renal arteriogram: X-ray of the arteries of the kidney.

Renal cell carcinoma: a type of kidney cancer.

Renal cysts: Abnormal fluid-filled sacs in the kidney that range in size from microscopic to much larger.

Renal osteodystrophy: Weak bones caused by poorly working kidneys.

Renal pelvis: The area of the kidney into which the urine formed by the kidneys is excreted before it drains down the ureters to the bladder.

Renal tubular acidosis: A defect in the kidneys that hinders their normal excretion of acids.

Renal vein thrombosis: blood clots in the vessels that carries blood away from the kidney.

Renal: Refers to the kidneys.

Renin: A hormone made by the kidneys that helps regulate the volume of fluid in the body and blood pressure.

Saline: A salt solution containing sodium and chloride.

Sodium: A mineral found in the body that helps regulate the fluid content in the body.

Stroke: Refers to inability of the brain to function normally resulting in physical weakness or paralysis.

Substituted judgment: Judgment (an educated guess) of what an individual would want under given circumstances based upon knowledge of that individual's values, beliefs, and attitudes or upon statements the individual made about another individual under similar circumstances.

Surrogate: A term generally interchangeable with "proxy," and indicating a person authorized or appointed to act for another. In some jurisdictions "surrogate" and "proxy" may be defined differently in the law.

Terminal sedation: Purposeful drowsiness due to medication administered to a terminally ill patient for the purpose of total relief of symptoms. "Terminal sedation" is sometimes called "controlled sedation for refractory suffering."

Tissue typing: A laboratory procedure used to determine the degree of compatibility between the donor kidney and the recipient of the kidney transplant.

Toxins: Waste products in the blood or any substance that is toxic to the body.

Transfusion: The injection of fluid, especially blood or plasma, into a vein.

Transplant: Replacement of a diseased organ with a healthy one.

Treatment directive (living will, healthcare instruction directive): An advance healthcare directive that specifies goals of treatment or specific treatments that are desired or that should be omitted. Normally such a directive becomes operative only when the patient is no longer able to make decisions for him or herself. The traditional living will was a treatment directive intended to limit care, particularly life-sustaining treatment.

Ultrafiltration: The method used to remove excess fluids form the blood during dialysis.

Ultrasound: A technique that bounces safe, painless sound waves off organs to create an image of their structure.

Urea Reduction Ratio (URR): A blood test that compares the amount of blood urea nitrogen before and after dialysis to measure the effectiveness of the dialysis dose.

Urea: A waste product found in the blood and caused by the normal breakdown of protein in the liver.

Uremia/Uremic: A condition associated with the loss of kidney function and the buildup of urea in the blood.

Ureter: The tube that carries urine from the kidney to the bladder.

Urethra: The tube that carries urine from the bladder to the outside of the body.

Urinalysis: A test of a urine sample that can reveal many problems of the urinary system and other body systems. The sample may be observed for color, cloudiness, concentration; signs of drug use; chemical composition, including sugar; the presence of protein, blood cells, or germs; or other signs of disease.

Urinary tract infection (UTI): An illness caused by harmful bacteria growing in the urinary tract.

Urinary tract: The system that takes wastes from the blood and carries them out of the body in the form of urine. The urinary tract includes the kidneys, renal pelvises, ureters, bladder and urethra.

Urinate: To release urine from the bladder to the outside; to void.

Urine: Liquid waste product filtered from the blood by the kidneys.

Urologist: A surgeon primarily concerned with the diagnosis and surgical treatment of disorders of the urinary system.

Values history: A series of questions intended to elicit the beliefs, values, health and treatment preferences of an individual. See Appendix G.

Vasculitis: Inflammation of the blood vessel walls.

Vein: A vessel carrying blood to the heart.

Vesicoureteral reflux: An abnormal condition in which urine backs up into the ureters, and occasionally into the kidneys, raising the risk of infection and kidney scarring.

Vitamin A: A fat-soluble vitamin found in egg yolk, fish-liver oils, liver, butter, cheese and many vegetables.

Vitamin B complex: An important group of water-soluble vitamins isolated from liver, yeast and other sources that includes thiamin, riboflavin, niacin, niacinimide, the vitamin B6 group, biotin, pantothenic acid, folic acid and others. The vitamin B complex group affects growth, appetite, lactation, and the gastrointestinal, nervous and endocrine systems.

Vitamin B12: Found primarily in animal products; essential for red blood cell formation.

Vitamin C: Ascorbic acid, found in citrus fruits and vegetables; aids in growth and prevents diseases such as scurvy.

Vitamin D: A fat-soluble vitamin found in milk products and from exposure to sunlight; necessary for the absorption of calcium and phosphorus; valuable in the formation of bones and teeth.

Vitamin E: A fat-soluble vitamin necessary in the body for reproduction and muscular development that is found in whole grains and vegetables.

Vitamin K: Found in green vegetables; important for the normal clotting of blood.

Vitamin: An organic substance that occurs in natural foods and is necessary in trace amounts for normal metabolic functioning of the body.

Void: To urinate, empty the bladder.

White blood cells: Blood cells in the body that destroy bacteria and foreign matter in the bloodstream.

Appendices

Appendix A
Blood Tests

Abbreviation	Type of Test	Reason for Test
Al	Aluminum	A trace metal. High blood levels suggest aluminum intoxication and may require chelation therapy because aluminum overload may cause brain dysfunction or bone disease.
Alb.	Albumin	Protein substance that helps hold fluid in blood vessels.
Alk Phos	Alkaline Phosphatase	An enzyme (a type of protein) in the liver and in bone; elevated levels may indicate liver or bone disease.
BUN	Blood Urea Nitrogen	Urea; byproduct of protein metabolism, indicator of levels of waste products in the blood, diet protein intake and the effectiveness of dialysis.
Ca	Calcium	Needed for bone-building; abnormal levels may be due to too much or too little calcium being deposited in bones or being absorbed from the diet.
Chol	Cholesterol	Fatty substance in blood; abnormal levels may lead to heart and blood vessel disease. Low levels indicate malnutrition.
Cl	Chloride	An essential element of blood that rises when bicarbonate falls.

Creat or Cr	Creatinine	A normal breakdown product of muscles that is removed by the kidneys and dialysis. Levels are monitored to determine the correct amount of dialysis.
Fe	Iron	Needed for red blood cells to be produced normally and to carry oxygen. Low levels indicate a need for iron therapy. High levels occur when there is an excess of iron in the body, but also when there is an acute inflammation in the body.
Ferritin	—	A protein that binds iron in the body.
Glu	Glucose	Blood sugar, which is high in diabetics, and most commonly is low when too much medication (insulin or oral hypoglycemic) is given to a diabetic.
HB$_s$Ag	Hepatitis B Surface Antigen	Test for current infection with (serum) Hepatitis B and for contagiousness.
Anti-HB$_s$	Hepatitis B Surface Antibody	Test for prior infection or immunity to Hepatitis B.
HCO3	Bicarbonate	A base, and, thus, indirectly, a test of acidity in the blood.
Hct	Hematocrit	Percentage of the blood that is red blood cells; low levels indicate anemia.
Hgb	Hemoglobin	The molecule within RBCs, which contains iron and which transports the oxygen and carbon dioxide. A low level indicates anemia and/or iron deficiency.

1,25(OH)$_2$, D$_3$	Calcitriol	The active form of Vitamin D (activated by the liver and by the kidneys), which has also been produced by pharmaceutical firms to be used as a medication.
K	Potassium	An essential element of the blood and especially of the fluid inside cells; abnormal levels (both high and low) could adversely affect the heart and cause muscle weakness.
LDH	Lactic Dehydrogenase	An enzyme; elevations may indicate general muscle damage, or increased destruction of red blood cells.
Mg	Magnesium	An element similar to calcium, which is predominantly inside cells and important to their function.
Na	Sodium	An essential element of blood and of the fluid outside cells; lower levels can cause muscle cramping; high levels cause excessive thirst, and lead to edema and hypertension.
P or PO$_4$	Phosphate	Elevated levels indicate excessive intake or failure to comply with phosphate binding medications or excessive parathyroid hormone.
Plts	Platelets	Small cells in the blood that help the blood to clot.
PTH	Parathyroid Hormone	A hormone produced in the parathyroid glands. High levels may cause bone disease.

Abbreviation	Name	Description
RBC	Red Blood Cells or Erythrocytes	The number of red blood cells that carry oxygen to the tissues and carbon dioxide from the tissues to the lungs. Normally, RBCs have a life span of 120 days.
Retics	Reticulocytes	Young, red blood cells. If a high percentage of red blood cells are reticulocytes, this is evidence of active red blood cell formation.
SGOT	Serum Glutamic Oxaloacetic Transaminase	An enzyme; elevations usually indicate liver damage, though this enzyme also rises acutely if there is muscle injury, as in a heart attack.
SGPT	Serum Glutamic Pyruvic	An enzyme; elevations indicate liver damage.
T. Bili.	Total Bilirubin	Waste product which must be removed by liver through the bile ducts and increases with liver or gall bladder disease.
T.P.	Total Protein	Amount of protein in blood, mostly albumin and globulin.
Transferrin	Transferrin	A protein that transports iron in the blood (before it is incorporated in Hgb) and that increases when iron is deficient.
Uric Acid	Uric Acid	A waste product from protein in the diet that should be removed to prevent gouty arthritis and kidney stones.
WBC	White Blood Cells	Cells that fight infection. High levels usually indicate infection, and very low levels indicate susceptibility to infection.

Adapted from *Understanding Your New Life With Dialysis*, Edith T. Overley, M.A., and Terry D. Oberley, M.D., Ph.D., second edition, 1978. Courtesy of Charlles C. Thomas, Publisher, Springfield, Illinois.

Appendix B
Food Lists

Foods are grouped under the following main headings: meats and meat substitutes, dairy products, breads and cereals, fruits, vegetables and miscellaneous. An average nutrient value of protein, sodium, potassium and calories has been established for each group.

ABBREVIATIONS

c	= cup	K	= potassium
CA	= calcium	lge	= large
CAL	= calories	Low Sod	= Low Sodium
CHO	= carbohydrate	med	= medium
ck	= cooked	mEq	= milliequivalent
cnd	= canned	mg	= milligram
diam	= diameter	NA	= sodium
froz	= frozen	oz	= ounce
gm	= gram	P	= phosphorus

PRO	= protein		
sm	= small		
sw	= sweetened		
	(canned in syrup)		
Tbsp	= tablespoon		
tsp	= teaspoon		
tr	= trace		
unsw	= unsweetened		
"	= inch		

LOW SODIUM PROTEIN LIST

AVERAGES: Calories: 60 Protein: 8 gm Sodium: 30 mg Potassium: 100 mg Calcium: 10 mg Phosphorus: 70 mg

FOOD ITEM	HOUSEHOLD MEASURE	gm	CAL	gm PRO	gm FAT	gm CHO	mg CA	mg P	mg NA	mg K
Beef brisket	1 oz.	28	69	8	4	0	2	68	20	81
Beef chuck roast	1 oz.	28	79	9	5	0	3	68	18	75
Beef rib roast	1 oz.	28	100	7	8	0	3	49	18	84
Beef round	1 oz.	28	60	9	3	0	1	76	14	86
Beef loin	1 oz.	28	61	8	3	0	2	59	17	96
Beef, ground, x-lean	1 oz.	28	48	7	2	0	2	58	20	97
Cottage cheese, 1% milk fat	1/4 c.		41	7	1	2	34	76	229	49
Chicken, no skin	1 oz.	28	53	7	2	0	3	54	21	64
Chicken, canned	1 oz.	28	59	7	2	0	4	43	38	43
Duck, no skin	1 oz.	28	56	7	3	0	3	57	18	71
Egg, whole	1 lg	50	74	6	5	trace	27	96	70	67
Egg whites	2	66	34	7	trace	trace	5	10	110	108
Lamb	1 oz.	8	73	7	5	0	5	55	20	90
Pork, fresh	1 oz.	28	70	8	4	0	5	69	17	116
Rabbit	1 oz.	28	56	8	2	0	5	75	13	109
Turkey, no skin	1 oz.	28	44	8	1	0	5	61	18	85
Veal	1 oz.	28	52	7	2	0	8	61	27	91
Venison	1 oz.	28	42	8	1	0	7	78	16	111

LOW SODIUM PROTEIN LIST (continued)

AVERAGES: Calories: 60 Protein: 8 gm Sodium: 30 mg Potassium: 100 mg Calcium: 10 mg Phosphorus: 70 mg

FOOD ITEM	HOUSEHOLD MEASURE	gm	CAL	gm PRO	m FAT	gm CHO	mg CA	mg P	mg NA	mg K
ORGAN MEATS:										
Beef heart	1 oz.	28	30	5	1	trace	2	60	28	81
Beef kidney	1 oz.	28	28	5	1	trace	4	73	52	74
Beef liver	1 oz.	28	38	6	2	1	1	108	19	88
Beef tongue	1 oz.	28	64	4	5	1	2	38	20	89
Chicken gizzard	1/4 c.	36	32	6	1	0	4	53	23	35
Chicken liver	1/4 c.	35	42	6	2	trace	3	104	25	81
Pork liver	1 oz.	28	38	6	1	1	3	82	25	77
Turkey giblets	1/4 c.	36	46	7	2	1	3	79	31	114
SEAFOOD:										
Bass, baked	1 oz.	28	41	7	1	0	29	79	26	129
Clams, steamed	3 med.	42	63	11	1	2	39	144	48	268
Cod, broiled	1 oz.	28	30	6	trace	0	4	39	22	69
Haddock, broiled	1 oz.	28	32	7	trace	0	12	68	25	113
Salmon, Sole/Flounder, broiled	1 oz.	28	58, 33	6, 7	4, trace	0	4, 5	71, 82	17, 30	109, 97
Halibut	1 oz.	28	40	8	1	0	17	81	20	163
Lobster	1/4 c.	36	51	10	1	1	23	82	82	75
Oysters, raw	3 med.	47	35	2	1	2	18	39	75	52
Scallops, steamed	3 lg.	28	31	7	trace	0	32	95	74	133
Shrimp, boiled	5 lg.	28	27	6	trace	0	11	38	50	62
Tuna, canned LS	1/4 c.	40	46	10	trace	0	4	65	20	95

HIGH SODIUM PROTEIN LIST

AVERAGES: Calories: 60 Protein: 8 gm Sodium: 180 mg Potassium: 100 mg Calcium: 20 mg Phosphorus: 80 mg

FOOD ITEM	HOUSEHOLD MEASURE	gm	CAL	gm PRO	m FAT	gm CHO	mg CA	mg P	mg NA	mg K
Chicken, canned	1 oz.	28	57	5	4	1	0	31	265	173
Cottage cheese, reg.	1/4 c.	57	59	7	3	2	34	75	231	48
Cottage cheese, LF	1/4 c.	57	51	8	1	2	39	85	229	54
Salmon, canned-oil	1/4 c.	40	56	8	2	0	85	132	222	130
Tuna, canned-oil	1/4 c.	40	79	12	3	0	5	124	142	83
Tuna, canned-water	1/4 c.	40	46	10	trace	0	4	65	135	95
Turkey breast, smkd.	1 oz.	28	28	5	1	1	3	73	257	73
Turkey, canned	1 oz.	28	46	7	2	0	3	45	131	63
Turkey roll	1 oz.	28	42	5	2	1	9	48	166	77

SUPPLEMENTAL PROTEIN LIST

Directions for use: These foods contribute a significant amount of potassium and phosphorus and are sources of low biological value protein, and should be calculated into a Patient diet on an individual basis.

AVERAGES: Calories: 120 Protein: 8 gm Sodium: 10 mg Potassium: 30 mg Calcium: 35 mg Phosphorus: 130 mg

FOOD ITEM	HOUSEHOLD MEASURE	gm	CAL	gm PRO	m FAT	gm CHO	mg CA	mg P	mg NA	mg K
Beans, cooked without salt:										
Blackeyed peas	1/2 c.	86	114	8	trace	20	23	120	1	305
Garbanzo beans	1/2 c.	82	134	7	2	22	40	138	6	239
Kidney beans	1/2 c.	89	112	7	trace	20	25	126	2	357
Lentils	2/3 c.	131	152	12	1	26	25	235	3	482
Peanut butter*	2 Tbs.	32	190	8	16	6	12	118	5	214
*unsalted										

DAIRY LIST

AVERAGES: Calories: Varies Protein: 4 gm Sodium: 85 mg Potassium: 190 mg Calcium: 150 mg Phosphorus: 120 mg

FOOD ITEM	HOUSEHOLD MEASURE	gm	CAL	gm PRO	m FAT	gm CHO	mg CA	mg P	mg NA	mg K
MILK:										
Whole milk	1/2 c.	122	73	4	4	6	125	102	52	162
LF milk, 2%	1/2 c.	122	61	4	2	6	135	112	57	171
LF milk, hi pro	1/2 c.	123	69	5	2	7	176	138	73	224
Non-fat milk	1/2 c.	123	42	4	trace	6	111	91	54	119
Buttermilk	1/2 c.	123	49	4	1	6	142	109	129	185
Calci-milk	1/2 c.	122	45	4	trace	6	200	118	62	190
Choc. milk, whole	1/2 c.	125	104	4	4	13	140	126	75	209
Choc. milk, LF	1/2 c.	125	79	4	1	13	144	129	76	213
Cocoa, mix + water	1 c.	240	132	2	1	28	53	105	170	235
Cream, half & half	1/2 c.	121	157	4	14	5	127	115	50	157
Eggnog, no ETOH	1/2 c.	127	171	5	10	17	165	138	69	210
Evap. milk, whole	1/4 c.	63	84	4	5	6	164	128	67	191
Evap. milk, skim	1/4 c.	64	50	5	trace	7	186	129	74	212
Goat's milk, skim	1/2 c.	122	84	5	5	5	163	135	61	249
LactAid, LF	1/2 c.	122	60	4	2	6	120	118	62	190
LactAid, skim	1/2 c.	122	45	4	trace	6	130	96	62	190
Powd/dry NF milk	2 Tbs.	15	54	5	trace	8	189	145	80	269

DAIRY LIST (continued)

AVERAGES: Calories: Varies Protein: 4 gm Sodium: 85 mg Potassium: 190 mg Calcium: 150 mg Phosphorus: 120 mg

FOOD ITEM	HOUSEHOLD MEASURE	gm	CAL	gm PRO	gm FAT	gm CHO	mg CA	mg P	mg NA	mg K
PUDDING:										
D'zerta, w/skim	1/2 c.	150	67	4	0	12	120	100	67	190
Mix, not instant	1/2 c.	130	463	2	trace	110	64	16	295	23
Cup, Kraft Jell-O brand										
Vanilla, ready to eat	4 oz.	113	104	2	trace	23	86	115	241	123
Pudd. pop, Jello	2 bars	108	150	4	4	26	128	64	130	190
YOGURT:										
LF, fruited	1/2 c.	123	121	5	1	23	169	134	65	217
LF, vanilla	1/2 c.	123	104	6	2	17	209	165	81	268
LF, plain	1/2 c.	123	77	6	2	9	224	176	86	287
Non-fat, plain	1/2 c.	123	69	7	trace	9	244	192	94	312
FROZEN DESSERTS:										
Fudgsicle	1 bar	73	91	4	trace	19	129	99	55	173
Ice cream, vanilla	3/4 c.	161	400	6	26	36	188	169	98	252
Ice milk, hard	3/4 c.	100	138	4	4	22	132	97	79	199
Soft-serve ice milk	1/2 c.	88	195	4	11	20	115	102	54	156

CHEESE LIST

AVERAGES: Calories: Varies Protein: 4 gm Sodium: 85 mg Potassium: 190 mg Calcium: 150 mg Phosphorus: 120 mg

FOOD ITEM	HOUSEHOLD MEASURE	gm	CAL	gm PRO	m FAT	gm CHO	mg CA	mg P	mg NA	mg K
NATURAL CHEESES:										
Bleu cheese	1/2 oz.	14	50	3	4	trace	75	55	198	36
Brie cheese	1/2 oz.	14	47	3	4	trace	26	27	89	22
Cheddar cheese	1/2 oz.	14	57	4	5	trace	102	73	88	14
Gouda cheese	1/2 oz.	14	50	4	5	trace	99	77	116	17
Colby cheese	1/2 oz.	14	56	3	5	trace	97	65	86	18
Gruyere cheese	1/2 oz.	14	99	4	5	trace	143	86	48	11
Jack cheese	1/2 oz.	14	53	3	4	0	106	63	76	12
Mozzarella, skim	1/2 oz.	14	21	4	0	trace	135	92	104	15
Swiss cheese	1/2 oz.	14	54	4	4	1	112	80	27	11

BREAD AND STARCH LIST

AVERAGES: Calories: 90 Protein: 2 gm Sodium: 160 mg Potassium: 35 mg Calcium: 20 mg Phosphorus: 35 mg

FOOD ITEM	HOUSEHOLD MEASURE	gm	CAL	gm PRO	m FAT	gm CHO	mg CA	mg P	mg NA	mg K
Roll, parkerhouse	1	24	75	2	1	13	9	21	127	23
Tortilla, corn	1	24	53	1	1	11	42	75	39	37
Tortilla, flour	1 (6")	46	150	4	3	26	58	57	220	60
Taco shell	1 (8")	51	146	4	3	25	97	50	249	50
Waffle, frozen	1	38	95	2	3	15	84	152	284	46
Danish (chesse)	1	91	353	6	25	27	70	80	319	116
Donut, cake (small)	1	60	250	3	12	34	128	97	204	64
Donut, raised	1	30	124	2	8	11	11	23	70	24
DESSERTS:										
Cake, yellow (no frosting)	2" x 2"	48	173	3	7	25	70	56	165	44
Cake, pound	1 sl.	30	116	2	6	15	11	41	119	36
Cupcake, iced	1	43	131	2	2	29	15	79	178	96
Butter cookies	6	30	140	2	6	21	9	31	105	32
Choc chip cookies	2	20	96	1	5	13	5	22	63	27
Shortbread	4 pcs.	32	161	2	8	21	11	35	146	32
Sugar cookies	4	32	142	2	5	22	25	33	102	24
Sugar wafers	4	60	287	3	13	41	13	48	214	38
Vanilla wafers	10	60	284	3	12	43	15	38	184	64
Animal crackers	10	25	112	2	3	19	11	29	98	25

BREAD AND STARCH LIST (continued)

AVERAGES: Calories: 90 Protein: 2 gm Sodium: 160 mg Potassium: 35 mg Calcium: 20 mg Phosphorus: 35 mg

FOOD ITEM	HOUSEHOLD MEASURE	gm	CAL	gm PRO	m FAT	gm CHO	mg CA	mg P	mg NA	mg K
Arrowroot crackers	6	29	131	2	4	22	13	34	116	29
Brownie	1 sm.	22	89	1	4	14	6	22	69	33
SNACKS:										
Corn chips	1 oz.	28	153	2	9	16	36	52	179	40
Reg. tortilla chips	1 oz.	28	142	2	7	18	44	58	150	56
Saltines	8	24	104	2	3	17	29	25	312	31
Soda crackers	8	23	100	2	3	16	5	20	250	27
Oyster crackers	30	30	130	3	4	21	36	32	391	38
Ritz crackers	8	27	133	2	6	17	40	81	210	25
CEREALS:										
Captain Crunch	1 c.	27	108	1	2	23	4	45	202	54
Cocoa Krispies	1 c.	41	157	1	1	36	53	41	253	67
Corn Chex	1 c.	30	112	2	trace	26	100	22	288	25
Cornflakes	1 c.	28	101	2	trace	24	2	14	203	25
Fruity Pebbles	1 c.	36	144	1	1	32	2	21	210	40
Kix	1 c.	23	85	1	trace	19	113	36	201	26
Rice Krispies	1 c.	26	95	2	trace	23	4	33	255	35
Sugar Frosted Flakes	1 c.	41	152	1	trace	37	2	14	198	30
Trix	1 c.	30	117	1	1	27	100	20	194	17

BREAD AND STARCH LIST (continued)

AVERAGES: Calories: 90 Protein: 2 gm Sodium: 5 mg Potassium: 35 mg Calcium: 10 mg Phosphorus: 35 mg

FOOD ITEM	HOUSEHOLD MEASURE	gm	CAL	gm PRO	m FAT	gm CHO	mg CA	mg P	mg NA	mg K
BREADS:										
Rice wafers	2	18	70	2	0	16	—	—	20	50
Matzo	1 pc.	28	111	3	trace	23	4	25	1	31
Low sodium bread	1 sl.	25	67	2	1	12	27	24	7	30
Ladyfingers	2	22	80	2	2	13	10	38	32	25
Melba toast	4 pcs.	20	78	2	1	15	19	39	166	40
Popcorn (no salt, no oil)	1 c.	14	73	1	4	8	1	35	0	32
Ice cream cone (sugar)	1	10	40	1	trace	8	4	10	32	15
CEREALS: (Cooked without salt)										
Corn grits	1/2 c.	121	71	2	trace	16	4	13	2	25
Cream of rice	1/2 c.	122	63	1	trace	14	4	21	1	24
Cream of wheat	1/2 c.	126	63	2	trace	13	56	40	73	23
Farina	1/2 c.	117	56	2	trace	12	5	14	2	15
Oatmeal	1/2 c.	117	74	3	1	13	9	89	1	66
Malt-O-Meal	1/2 c.	126	61	2	trace	13	2	12	1	16
LS Cornflakes	1 c.	26	100	2	trace	22	10	12	2	18
LS Rice Krispies	1 c.	28	114	2	trace	26	19	29	3	22
Frosted MiniWheats	1/2 c.	28	95	3	trace	22	9	81	2	95
Puffed Rice	1 c.	14	56	1	trace	13	1	14	0	16

BREAD AND STARCH LIST (continued)

AVERAGES: Calories: 90 Protein: 2 gm Sodium: 5 mg Potassium: 35 mg Calcium: 10 mg Phosphorus: 35 mg

FOOD ITEM	HOUSEHOLD MEASURE	gm	CAL	gm PRO	m FAT	gm CHO	mg CA	mg P	mg NA	mg K
Puffed Wheat	1 c.	12	44	2	trace	10	3	43	0	42
Shredded Wheat	1 biscuit	23	78	3	1	18	10	82	3	85
STARCHES: (Cooked without salt)										
Macaroni, cooked	1/2 c.	70	99	3	trace	20	5	38	1	22
Noodles, cooked	1/2 c.	80	106	4	1	20	10	55	6	22
Brown rice, cooked	1/2 c.	98	109	2	1	23	10	75	1	77
White rice, cooked	1/2 c.	93	121	2	trace	27	3	34	0	27
Spaghetti, cooked	1/2 c.	70	99	3	trace	20	5	38	1	22
White flour	2 Tbs.	16	52	2	trace	12	2	17	0	17

LOW POTASSIUM FRUIT LIST

AVERAGES: Calories: 60 Protein: <1 gm Sodium: 5 mg Potassium: 100 mg Calcium: 15 mg Phosphorus: 13 mg

FOOD ITEM	HOUSEHOLD MEASURE	gm	CAL	gm PRO	m FAT	gm CHO	mg CA	mg P	mg NA	mg K
FRUITS WITHOUT ADDED SUGAR:										
Acerola	10 ea.	48	15	trace	trace	4	6	5	3	70
Apple, dried	4 rings	26	62	trace	trace	17	4	10	22	115
Apple, fresh	1 sm.	106	55	trace	trace	15	6	12	1	113
Applesauce	1/2 c.	122	52	trace	trace	14	4	9	2	92
Blackberries	1/2 c.	72	31	1	trace	7	21	16	1	117
Blueberries	1/2 c.	73	44	1	trace	11	4	9	1	56
Boysenberries	1/2 c.	66	33	1	trace	8	18	18	1	92
Carissa, fresh	2 ea.	40	25	trace	1	5	4	3	1	104
Cherries, sour red, water-pack	1/2 c.	122	44	1	trace	11	13	12	9	120
Crabapples, sliced	1/2 c.	55	42	trace	trace	11	10	8	1	107
Cranberries, raw	1 c.	95	44	trace	trace	12	8	12	2	81
Fig, dried	1	34	21	trace	trace	5	14	6	1	57
Fig, fresh	1	50	37	trace	trace	10	18	7	1	116
Fig, canned water	1/2 c.	124	66	1	trace	17	35	12	1	128
Fruit cocktail in water	1/2 c.	119	38	1	trace	10	6	13	5	111
Fruit salad, canned in water	1/2 c.	123	37	trace	trace	10	9	11	4	96
Gooseberries raw	1/2 c.	75	33	1	trace	8	19	20	1	149
Grapes, fresh	1/2 c.	80	55	1	trace	14	8	16	2	153
Kumquats	4 ea.	76	54	1	1	12	47	14	8	141

LOW POTASSIUM FRUIT LIST (continued)

AVERAGES: Calories: 60 Protein: <1 gm Sodium: 5 mg Potassium: 100 mg Calcium: 15 mg Phosphorus: 13 mg

FOOD ITEM	HOUSEHOLD MEASURE	gm	CAL	gm PRO	m FAT	gm CHO	mg CA	mg P	mg NA	mg K
Lemon, no peel	1 med.	58	17	1	trace	5	15	9	1	80
Lime, no peel	1 ea.	67	15	trace	trace	6	9	9	1	78
Loganberries	1/2 c.	74	40	1	trace	10	19	19	1	107
Loquats, fresh	5 ea.	68	32	trace	trace	8	11	18	1	181
Lychees, fresh	8 ea.	77	51	1	trace	13	4	24	1	131
Mulberries	1/2 c.	70	30	1	trace	7	27	27	7	136
Oheloberries	1 c.	140	39	1	trace	10	10	14	1	53
Passion fruit	2 ea.	36	36	1	trace	8	4	24	10	126
Peaches, canned in water	1/2 c.	122	29	1	trace	7	2	12	4	121
Pears, canned in water	1/2 c.	122	35	trace	trace	10	5	9	2	65
Persimmon (native)	1 ea.	25	32	trace	trace	8	7	7	0	78
Pineapple canned in water	1/2 c.	123	39	1	trace	10	18	5	1	156
Pineapple, fresh	1/2 c.	78	37	trace	trace	10	10	6	1	89
Pitanga, fresh	1/2 c.	87	29	1	trace	6	8	6	3	89
Plum, fresh	1 med.	66	30	trace	trace	8	4	10	0	104
Raspberries	1/2 c.	62	32	1	trace	7	15	11	1	93
Roselle, fresh	1 c.	57	28	1	trace	6	123	18	3	119
Strawberries, sliced	1/2 c.	83	27	1	trace	6	13	21	1	127
Tamarind, fresh	10 ea.	20	48	1	trace	13	15	20	6	126
Tangerine, fresh	1 med.	84	37	1	trace	9	12	23	1	132
Watermelon	1/16 sl.	286	68	2	trace	22	20	31	3	320

LOW POTASSIUM FRUIT LIST (continued)

AVERAGES: Calories: 60 Protein: <1 gm Sodium: 5 mg Potassium: 100 mg Calcium: 15 mg Phosphorus: 13 mg

FOOD ITEM	HOUSEHOLD MEASURE	gm	CAL	gm PRO	m FAT	gm CHO	mg CA	mg P	mg NA	mg K
FRUIT JUICE - NO SUGAR ADDED:										
Acerola juice, fresh	1/2 c.	121	28	trace	trace	6	12	11	4	117
Apple juice	1/2 c.	124	58	trace	trace	14	9	9	4	148
Lemon juice	1/2 c.	122	31	trace	0	11	9	7	1	151
Lime juice	1/2 c.	246	66	1	trace	22	22	17	2	263

MODERATE POTASSIUM FRUIT LIST

AVERAGES: Calories: 60 Protein: <1 gm Sodium: 5 mg Potassium: 200 mg Calcium: 15 mg Phosphorus: 17 mg

FOOD ITEM	HOUSEHOLD MEASURE	gm	CAL	gm PRO	m FAT	gm CHO	mg CA	mg P	mg NA	mg K
FRUITS WITHOUT ADDED SUGAR:										
Apricot, fresh	2 ea.	70	34	1	trace	8	9	16	1	181
Apricot, canned in water	1/2 c.	114	25	1	trace	6	9	18	12	175
Apricot, dried	4 halves	14	12	trace	trace	3	3	4	1	58
Carambola, fresh	1 ea.	127	42	1	trace	10	5	20	3	207
Cherries, sweet, fresh	1/2 c.	73	46	1	trace	12	9	15	0	161
Cherries, sweet, canned	1/2 c.	124	57	1	trace	15	14	19	1	162
Dates, domestic	4 ea.	33	94	trace	trace	25	13	21	1	218
Elderberries	1/2 c.	73	53	1	trace	13	28	28	4	203
Grapefruit, fresh	1/2	128	41	1	trace	10	15	10	0	178
Grapefruit, canned	1/2 c.	122	44	1	trace	11	18	12	2	161
Mandarin oranges	1/2 c.	98	43	1	trace	11	14	10	1	153
Peach, fresh	1 sm.	79	31	1	trace	8	5	11	0	171
Pear, fresh	1 med.	166	96	1	trace	26	15	18	2	198
Plum, canned	1/2 c.	125	51	trace	trace	15	9	16	1	157
Prickly pear	1 ea.	103	42	1	1	10	58	25	5	227
Prunes, dried	3 ea.	25	60	1	trace	16	11	17	1	184
Quince, fresh	1 ea.	92	52	trace	trace	14	10	16	4	181
Raisins	2 Tbs.	21	63	1	trace	17	11	21	2	157

MODERATE TO HIGH POTASSIUM FRUIT JUICE LIST

AVERAGES: Calories: 60 Protein: 60 Protein: <1 gm Sodium: 5 mg Potassium: 200 mg Calcium: 15 mg Phosphorus: 17 mg

FOOD ITEM	HOUSEHOLD MEASURE	gm	CAL	gm PRO	m FAT	gm CHO	mg CA	mg P	mg NA	mg K
FRUIT JUICE - NO SUGAR ADDED:										
Grapefruit juice	1/2 c.	124	48	1	trace	11	11	19	1	200
Orange juice	1/2 c.	124	56	1	trace	13	14	21	1	248
Orange-grapefruit juice	1/2 c.	124	53	1	trace	13	10	17	4	195
Pineapple juice	1/2 c.	125	70	trace	trace	17	21	10	1	168

HIGH POTASSIUM FRUIT LIST

Note: These fruits are very high in potassium and should be used only when approved by the dietician.

FOOD ITEM	HOUSEHOLD MEASURE	gm	CAL	gm PRO	m FAT	gm CHO	mg CA	mg P	mg NA	mg K
Avocado	1/4	43	72	1	7	4	6	23	3	219
Banana	1 med.	113	105	1	trace	27	6	26	1	422
Breadfruit, fresh	1/4 sm.	96	99	1	trace	26	16	29	2	470
Currants, dried	1/4 c.	36	102	1	trace	27	31	45	3	321
Guava, common	1 ea.	90	45	1	1	11	18	23	2	256
Kiwifruit, fresh	1 ea.	76	46	1	trace	11	26	26	2	237
Mango, fresh	1 med.	207	135	1	trace	35	21	23	4	323
Melon, cantaloupe	1/4	204	69	2	trace	17	18	31	33	545
Melon, casaba	1/10	164	46	2	trace	11	18	8	15	298
Melon, honeydew	1/10	160	58	1	trace	15	10	18	29	365
Nectarine	1 ea.	136	60	1	trace	14	8	35	0	273
Orange, fresh	1 sm.	96	45	1	trace	11	38	13	0	174
Papaya, fresh	1/2 ea.	152	59	1	trace	15	36	8	5	391
Persimmon, dried	1 ea.	34	93	trace	trace	65	9	28	1	273
Plantain, fresh	1/2 ea.	90	109	1	trace	29	3	30	4	447
Pomegranate, fresh	1	154	105	1	trace	26	5	12	5	399
Prune juice, canned	1/2 c.	128	91	1	trace	22	15	32	5	353
Prunes, canned	1/2 c.	117	123	1	trace	33	20	30	3	264
Pummelo, fresh	1/2 ea.	305	116	2	trace	29	12	52	3	658
Sapodilla, fresh	1 ea.	170	141	1	2	34	36	20	20	328
Soursop, fresh	1/2 ea.	313	206	3	1	53	44	84	44	869
Tamarind, pulp	1/2 c.	60	143	2	trace	38	44	68	17	377
Tangelo, fresh	1 med.	170	39	1	trace	9	27	20	2	296

LOW POTASSIUM VEGETABLE LIST

AVERAGES: Calories: 15 Protein: 1 gm Sodium: 20 mg Potassium: 100 mg Calcium: 20 mg Phosphorus: 18 mg

FOOD ITEM	HOUSEHOLD MEASURE	gm	CAL	gm PRO	m FAT	gm CHO	mg CA	mg P	mg NA	mg K
Amaranth, whole, raw	1/2 c.	14	3	trace	trace	1	30	7	3	86
Bamboo shoots	1/2 c.	76	21	2	1	4	10	45	3	405
Beans, Mung, raw	1/2 c.	104	359	25	trace	65	137	380	16	1290
Beans, snap, raw	1/2 c.	55	17	1	trace	4	20	21	3	115
Beans, snap, cooked	1/2 c.	63	22	1	trace	5	28	18	1	91
Broccoli, raw	1/2 c.	44	15	1	trace	3	21	29	15	139
Cabbage, Chinese	1/2 c.	35	5	1	trace	1	37	13	23	88
Cabbage, green, raw	1/2 c.	35	8	trace	trace	2	16	8	6	86
Cabbage, red, raw	1/2 c.	35	11	1	trace	3	16	11	9	85
Carrots, cooked	1/2 c.	73	27	trace	trace	6	26	23	43	140
Chicory root, raw	1/2 c.	45	33	1	trace	8	18	27	23	131
Cucumber, raw	1/2 c.	60	7	trace	trace	1	8	12	1	81
Dandelion, green, ckd	1/2 c.	53	17	1	trace	3	74	22	23	122
Eggplant, boiled	1/2 c.	50	17	trace	trace	4	3	7	0	61
Endive, raw	1/2 c.	25	4	trace	trace	1	13	7	6	79
Leeks, raw	1/2 c.	45	27	1	trace	6	36	16	9	80
Lettuce, iceberg	1/2 c.	28	3	trace	trace	1	6	6	2	42
Lettuce, romaine	1/2 c.	28	5	trace	trace	1	9	8	2	69
Mushrooms, raw	1/2 c.	35	8	1	trace	1	1	30	1	110
Mushroom, Shiitake	1/2 c.	73	40	1	trace	10	2	21	3	85
Mustard green, raw	1/2 c.	28	7	1	trace	1	29	12	7	99

LOW POTASSIUM VEGETABLE LIST (continued)

AVERAGES: Calories: 15 Protein: 1 gm Sodium: 20 mg Potassium: 100 mg Calcium: 20 mg Phosphorus: 18 mg

FOOD ITEM	HOUSEHOLD MEASURE	gm	CAL	gm PRO	m FAT	gm CHO	mg CA	mg P	mg NA	mg K
Mustard greens, cooked	1/2 c.	70	11	2	trace	1	52	29	11	141
Onions, raw	1/2 c.	80	34	1	trace	8	18	22	2	115
Pea pods, raw	1/2 c.	32	13	1	trace	2	14	17	1	63
Peas & Carrots, cooked	1/2 c.	80	38	2	trace	8	18	39	54	126
Pepper, sweet, raw	1/2 c.	46	9	trace	trace	2	5	9	1	81
Purslane, raw	1/2 c.	22	3	trace	trace	1	14	9	10	106
Radishes, raw	1/2 c.	58	9	trace	trace	2	14	12	23	135
Squash, summer	1/2 c.	57	9	1	trace	2	8	21	1	1488
Squash, winter	1/2 c.	58	20	1	trace	5	16	13	2	203
Squash, spaghetti	1/2 c.	51	16	trace	trace	3	12	6	9	55
Swamp cabbage	1/2 c.	28	5	1	trace	1	22	11	32	37
Turnips, boiled	1/2 c.	78	17	1	trace	4	26	20	12	138
Turnip greens, raw	1/2 c.	28	6	1	trace	1	32	7	5	23
Yambean (jicama)	1/2 c.	65	25	trace	trace	6	8	12	3	98

MODERATE TO HIGH POTASSIUM VEGETABLE LIST

AVERAGES: Calories: 40 Protein: 1 gm Sodium: 20 mg Potassium: 200 mg Calcium: 27 mg Phosphorus: 36 mg

FOOD ITEM	HOUSEHOLD MEASURE	gm	CAL	gm PRO	m FAT	gm CHO	mg CA	mg P	mg NA	mg K
Artichoke hearts	1/2 c.	84	42	3	trace	9	38	72	80	397
Asparagus, raw	4 spears	64	13	1	trace	2	15	33	1	129
Asparagus, cooked	4 spears	60	11	2	trace	1	11	29	2	103
Beets, cooked	1/2 c.	85	37	1	trace	8	14	32	65	269
Broccoli, cooked	1/2 c.	78	27	2	trace	6	31	52	32	229
Burdock root, cooked	1/2 c.	63	55	1	trace	13	31	58	3	225
Carrot, raw	1/2 c.	61	25	1	trace	6	20	21	342	195
Cauliflower, raw	1/2 c.	50	13	1	trace	3	11	22	15	152
Cauliflower, cooked	1/2 c.	62	14	1	trace	3	10	22	9	88
Celeriac, raw	1/2 c.	78	33	1	trace	7	34	90	78	234
Celery, raw	1/2 c.	60	8	trace	trace	2	24	14	48	146
Collards, cooked	1/2 c.	93	30	3	1	6	166	31	34	224
Corn, cooked	1/2 c.	82	89	3	1	21	2	84	14	204
Cress, raw	1/2 c.	25	8	1	trace	1	20	19	4	152
Dock (sorrel), raw	1/2 c.	67	15	1	trace	2	29	42	3	259
Kale, raw	1/2 c.	34	17	1	trace	3	45	19	14	150
Kale, cooked	1/2 c.	65	18	1	trace	4	47	18	15	148
Mixed veg., frozen	1/2 c.	87	56	3	trace	12	22	51	41	184
Okra, boiled	1/2 c.	80	18	2	trace	4	62	26	5	108
Parsley, raw	1/2 c.	30	11	1	trace	2	41	17	17	166
Peas, green, cooked	1/2 c.	80	67	4	trace	13	27	94	2	217

MODERATE TO HIGH POTASSIUM VEGETABLE LIST (continued)

AVERAGES: Calories: 40 Protein: 1 gm Sodium: 20 mg Potassium: 200 mg Calcium: 27 mg Phosphorus: 36 mg

FOOD ITEM	HOUSEHOLD MEASURE	gm	CAL	gm PRO	m FAT	gm CHO	mg CA	mg P	mg NA	mg K
Pepper, chili, raw	1 ea.	45	19	1	trace	4	6	19	4	145
Poi	1/2 c.	120	134	trace	trace	33	19	47	14	220
Potato, boiled, no skin	1/2 c.	78	67	1	trace	16	6	31	4	256
Pumpkin, cooked	1/2 c.	123	25	1	trace	6	18	37	1	232
Rutabaga, cooked	1/2 c.	85	33	1	trace	7	41	48	17	277
Spinach, raw	1/2 c.	15	3	trace	trace	1	15	7	12	84
Squash, summer, ckd.	1/2 c.	90	18	1	trace	4	24	35	1	173
Squash, zucchini	1/2 c.	120	19	1	trace	5	16	48	4	304
Succotash, cooked	1/2 c.	96	110	5	1	23	16	112	16	394
Tomato, raw	1/2 c.	90	16	1	trace	4	9	28	5	213
Tomato juice, no salt	1/2 c.	122	21	1	trace	5	12	22	12	278
Yam	1/2 c.	68	79	1	trace	19	10	33	5	254

NON-DAIRY PRODUCT LIST

FOOD ITEM	HOUSEHOLD MEASURE	gm	CAL	gm PRO	m FAT	gm CHO	mg CA	mg P	mg NA	mg K
Coffee Rich, liquid	1/4 c.	60	96	0.2	6	11	1	24	24	24
Coffee creamer substiute liquid (frozen) avg.	1/4 c.	60	82	0.1	6	7	5	38	47	115
Coffee whiteners, powder, average	2 Tbsp.	12	66	0.1	4	7	3	51	22	97
Cremora, Borden	2 Tbsp.	12	66	0.6	—	—	—	—	1	10
Dessert Whip, liquid	1/4 c.	60	164	0.6	11	—	—	—	40	20
Imitation sour cream	1/4 c.	58	120	1	6	4	2	26	59	93
Mocha Mix	1/4 c.	57	80	0.2	—	5	3	32	29	79
Party Pride Whip, liquid	2 Tbsp.	30	99	0.6	—	—	—	—	13	1
Poly Rich, liquid	1/4 c.	60	88	0.2	6	8	1	20	12	40
Rich's Whip Topping, whipped	1/2 c.	23	63	0	—	—	—	—	13	trace
DESSERTS:										
Gelatin, low Sodium, D'Zerta	1/2 c.	60	8	2.0	0	0	trace	trace	10	50
Gelatin, regular, flavored	1/2 c.	135	34	2	0	19	4	30	101	1
Mocha Mix, Frozen Dessert	3/4 c.	—	216	0.6	—	—	—	—	90	—
Sherbet	1/2 c.	96	135	1.1	2	29	51	37	44	90

BEVERAGE LIST

HOUSEHOLD FOOD ITEM	MEASURE	gm	CAL	gm PRO	m FAT	gm CHO	mg CA	mg P	mg NA	mg K
ALCOHOLIC BEVERAGES (use only if approved by Doctor):										
Beer, average	8 oz.	238	78	1	trace	4	12	31	10	59
Brandy, gin, vodka, rum, whiskey (80 proof)	3 oz.	83	193	—	—	0	—	3	1	2
Wine, sweet, dessert	4 oz.	118	183	trace	0	16	9	11	11	109
Wine, cooking	4 oz.	116	58	1	0	7	10	17	726	102
Wine, table, average	4 oz.	118	91	trace	0	4	9	15	7	99
BEVERAGES - Carbonated:										
Bubble-Up	8 oz.	240	90	0	—	22	—	—	33	9
Club soda	8 oz.	237	0	0	0	0	12	0	50	5
Cola	8 oz.	248	104	trace	0	27	7	32	10	2
Cola, sugar free average	8 oz.	237	2	trace	0	trace	9	21	14	0
Gingerale	8 oz.	244	33	0	0	21	7	0	17	2
Orange mixes	8 oz.	248	119	0	0	31	12	2	30	5
Root Beer	8 oz.	246	101	0	0	26	12	0	32	2
Pepsi Cola	8 oz.	240	110	0	—	28	—	—	28	9
Royal Crown Cola	8 oz.	240	110	0	—	28	—	—	22	4
Simba	8 oz.	240	90	0	0	22	—	—	40	2
Shasta, regular, avg.	8 oz.	240	110	0	—	27	—	—	25	4
Tab, sugar free	8 oz.	240	1	0	—	trace	—	—	33	9

BEVERAGE LIST (continued)

HOUSEHOLD FOOD ITEM	MEASURE	gm	CAL	gm PRO	m FAT	gm CHO	mg CA	mg P	mg NA	mg K
BEVERAGES - Coffee, Tea, Bouillon:										
Bouillon, low salt	1 cube	4	16	1	1	2	7	6	38	11
Bouillon, salted	1 cube	4	11	1	1	1	7	7	743	12
Coffee, regular, instant	1 level tsp.	0.9	2	trace	0	trace	1	3	0	32
Coffee, freeze dried, instant	1 level tsp.	0.9	1	trace	trace	trace	2	3	1	29
Coffee, instant, prepared from 2 gm powder	6 oz.	180	2	trace	trace	trace	4	7	2	65
Coffee, brewed weak	6 oz.	178	7	trace	1	0	2	5	2	35
Cranberry juice cocktail	8 oz.	253	116	1	trace	31	20	33	5	195
Grape juice	8 oz.	253	154	1	trace	38	23	28	8	334
Instant Breakfast	1 envelope	37	131	7	1	24	105	158	350	142
Kool Aid, sugar free	1 envelope	10	28	1	trace	8	16	8	1	—
Kool Aid, presweetened	1 envelope	10	38	0	0	10	3	3	0	0
Lemon juice	1 envelope	47	12	trace	0	4	2	3	1	58
Lemonade, frozen, diluted	8 oz.	240	107	0.1	trace	28	3	3	trace	40
Limeade, frozen, diluted	8 oz.	240	102	0.1	trace	27	3	3	trace	32
Orange Tang	8 oz.	25	92	0	0	25	92	42	2	48
Orange Tang, Tart	8 oz.	240	120	0	0	26	—	—	45	trace
Orange juice, concentrate	4 oz.	124	55	1	trace	13	12	14	1	236
Tea	8 oz.	237	2	0	0	1	0	2	7	88

The preceding food charts were provided courtesy of the California Dietetic Association, Los Angeles District.

Cookbooks

Cookbooks for Renal Patients

(Prices Subject to Change. Contact the publisher for the current price.)

TITLE	DESCRIPTION	COST	S&H	CHECK TO:
Carbohydrate and Sodium Controlled Recipes	For the diabetic HD pat ient & the PD patient who must control carbohydrate & saturated fat intake as well as sodium, potassium & fluid.	$7.50	$2.50	CRN of Calif/N.Nevada c/o Helen Christensen, RD 1542 Queenstown Ct. Sunnyvale, CA 94087
Cooking for David: A Culinary Dialysis Cookbook	Written by a renal dietitian and nurse/wife of dialysis patient. Discusses food selection, preparation and meal planning. Daily menus. 160 tested recipes with extensive nutrient analysis, NRD and Diabetic exchanges. information for locating and using special "dialysis-friendly" ingredients. 20% discount for group order of 5 or more books.	$24.00 CA: $1.86 tax	$6.00	Culinary Kidney Cooks PO Box 468 Huntington Beach, CA 92648 Or from: www.CulinaryKidneyCooks.com
Cooking the Renal Way	Variety of recipes plus sections on holiday menus and diabetic desserts. Includes nutrient analysis. Hemo & PD patients, includes diabetic. Updated 1993	$10.00	incl	Oregon CRN PO Box 29133 Portland, OR 97210-9133
Creative Cooking for Renal Diets / Creative Cooking for Renal Diabetic Diets	Includes recipes with nutrient analysis (not phos) and exchanges. Includes calorie boosters and fluid calculations..	$17.95	4.95	Senay Publishing PO Box 397 Chesterland, OH 44026 800-850-6987 Fax: 440-256-2237
Everyday Eating Cookbook	94 recipes with nutrient analysis and NRD exchanges. Includes Kids Kuisine, holiday ideas and high calorie beverages.	$7.50 $5.00 in IL	incl	NKF of Illinois 215 West Illinois, Unit 1C, Chicago, IL 60610 www.nkfi.org 312-321-1500
Food Power: A Nutrition Book For Kids with	Comprehensive information for feeding the picky eater, the overweight child & those on modified diets. Includes 29 recipes with nutrient analysis, dining	$22.50	incl	The Children's Hospital c/o Charlotte Stall, MA,RD
The Gourmet Renal Cookbook	100 page book features gourmet renal recipes and menus with nutrient analysis in food label format and NRD exchanges.	$14.95	incl	Lenox Hill Hospital c/o Linda Pino, RD Sol Goldman Renal Therapy Center 100 East 77th Street New York, NY 10021 212-434-3266
Kidney Friendly Comfort Foods: A Collection of s	Features 21 low-phosphorus recipes developed by a certified chef de cuisine and reviewed by a renal dietitian. cookbook features a foreword by celebrity chef Isaac Hayes.	Free	Free	Order from www.fosrenol.com 866-896-6152

DaVita Inc,   Copyrighted Material

Cookbooks

TITLE	DESCRIPTION	COST	S&H	CHECK TO:
The Kidney HELPER Cookbook	Middle Eastern recipes with nutrient analysis. 190 pp; Includes index of organizations, resources and on-line help.	$24.95	$4.00	Consumer Med Help Inc 2437 Bay Area Blvd #128 Houston, TX 77058 877-248-2331 Fax 281-576-8990 www.consumermedhelp.com/KHMECookbook.html
Now You're Cooking	129 pages, large print. Includes nutrient analysis and exchanges.	$18.00	$3.00	CRNNE The NKF of MA/RI/NH/VT 85 Astor Ave, Ste 2 Norwood, MA 02062 800-542-4001 www.kidneyhealth.org
Recipes for Eating Well with Chronic Kidney Disease	A cookbook developed by the National Kidney Foundation for dialysis patients and their families.	Free	Free	Download from Amgen website www.epogen.com
The Renal Gourmet	200 recipes incorporating herbs, spices & vinegars. Nutrient analysis included.	$21.00	incl	Emenar Inc. 13N625 Coombs Road Elgin, IL 60123 847-299-1226 www.kidney.cookbook.com
The Renal Patient's Guide to Good Eating	Over 200 pages of recipes from a kidney patient who is an avid cook; endorsed by a renal dietitian. Includes family meals, dining out and practical ideas	$36.95	$6.95	Charles C. Thomas, Publisher 2600 S. First Street PO Box 19265 Springfield IL 62794-9265 800-258-8980
Southern Comforts of Mississippi – A Cookbook For Patients & Their Families	Approximately 65 pages of recipes with nutrient analysis.	$10.00	incl	NKF of Mississippi PO Box 55802 Jackson, MS 39296-5802 601-981-3611 Fax: 601-981-3612
A Taste of Asia	Asian recipes for kidney patients. Includes nutrient analysis and glossary of ingredients	$10.00	incl	NKF No. California 611 Mission St, 3rd Floor San Francisco, CA 94105 415-543-3303 Fax: 415-543-3331

DaVita Inc,   Copyrighted Material

Appendix D
Weights and Measures

Dry Measurements	Approximate Conversion
1/4 teaspoon (tsp)	1 gram (gm)
1/2 tsp	2 gm
1 tsp	5 gm
3 tsp = 1 tablespoon (Tbsp)	15 gm
2 Tbsp = 1 ounce (oz)	30 gm
4 Tbsp = 1/4 cup = 2 oz	60 gm
16 Tbsp = 1 cup = 8 oz	240 gm

Liquid Measurements	Approximate Conversion to Metric System
2 tbsp = 1 ounce (oz)	30 milliliters (ml)
1 jigger = 1-1/2 oz	45 ml
1/4 cup = 2 oz	60 ml
1/3 cup = 2-2/3 oz	80 ml
1/2 cup = 4 oz	120 ml
2/3 cup = 5-1/3 oz	160 ml
3/4 cup = 6 oz	180 ml
1 cup = 8 oz	240 ml
2 cups = 16 oz = 1 pint	500 ml
4 cups = 32 oz = 1 quart	1000 ml = 1 liter

NOTE: 1 milliliter (ml) = 1 cubic centimeter (cc)

Appendix E
List of Medications

Type of Drug	Generic	Brand	Purpose
Analgesics	aspirin acetominophen ibuprofen naproxen	Ecotrin®, Bayer® Tylenol® Motrin® Naprosyn®, Aleve®	Helps relieve pain. Some may reduce fever.
Antibiotics	Cephalosporins Carbapenems Penicillins Macrolides Floroquinolones Vancomycin/linezolid Aminoglycosides		Stop the growth of bacteria or kill bacteria
Phosphate Binders	aluminum hydroxide	Alternagel® Amphojel® Alu-Tab® Alu-Cap® Aludrox®	Bind phosphate in intestine to help maintain proper calcium and phosphorus levels in the blood. (See calcium supplements)

Category	Generic	Brand	Action
	calcium carbonate	Tums®, Os-Cal®, Titralac®, Calci-Chew®, Caltrate®, Rolaids®, Nephro-Calci®	
	calcium acetate	PhosLo®	
	magaldrate	Riopan®	
	lanthanum carbonate	Fosrenol®	
	sevelamer hydrochloride	Renagel®	
Potassium Binders	Sodium Polystyrene sulfonate	Kayexalate®	Bind potassium in intestine to prevent elevated potassium level in blood
ACE Inhibitors	captopril	Capoten®	Lower blood pressure
	benazepril	Lotensin®	
	enalapril	Vasotec®	
	prinivil	Zestril®	
	fosinopril	Monopril®	
	ramipril	Altace®	
	perindopril	Aceon®	
	quinapril	Accupril®	
	moexipril	Univasc®	
	trandolapril	Mavik®	

Category	Generic	Brand	Action
Angiotensin II Receptor Blockers	losartan candesartan irbesartan temisartan valsartan	Cozaar® Atacand® Avapro® Micardis® Diovan®	Lower blood pressure
Diuretics (Thiazide)	hydrochlorothiazide Chlorthalidone Metolazone Indapamide Polythiazide	Hydrodiuril® Hygroton® Zaroxolyn® Lozol® Renese®	Lower blood pressure
Diuretics (Loop)	Furosemide Bumetanide Torsemide Ethacrynic acid	Lasix® Bumex® Demadex® Edecrin®	Lower blood pressure
K-sparing Diuretics	amiloride triamterene spironolactone eplerenone	Midamor® Dyrenium® Aldactone® Inspra®	Lower blood pressure

Calcium Channel Blockers	amlodipine	Norvasc®	Lower blood pressure
	felodipine	Plendil®	
	nifedipine	Procardia®	
	diltiazem	Cardizem®	
	verapamil	Calan®	
Alpha-adrenergic Blockers	doxazosin	Cardura®	Lower blood pressure
	prazosin	Minipress®	
	terazosin	Hytrin®	
Direct Vasodilators	hydralazine	Apresoline®	Lower blood pressure
	minoxidil	Loniten®	
Beta Blockers	acebutolol	Sectral®	Lower blood pressure
	atenolol	Tenormin®	
	betaxolol	Kerlone®	
	bisoprolol	Zebeta®	
	carteolol	Cartrol®	
	metoprolol	Lopressor®, Toprol XL®	
	nadolol	Cogard®	
	penbutolol	Levatol®	
	pindolol	Visken®	

Category	Generic	Brand	Description
	propranolol timolol carvedilol labetolol	Inderal® Berimol® Coreg® Normodyne®, Trandate®	
Calcium Supplements	calcium carbonate calcium acetate calcium citrate calcium chloride calcium gluconate	Tums®, Os-Cal®, Titralac®, Calci-Chew®, Caltrate®, Rolaids®, Nephro-Calci® PhosLo® Citracal® Calciject® Calcionate®, Neo-Calgluconate®	Increase the amount of calcium in the blood and body. Also function as phosphate binders if taken with meal (See phosphate binders)
Folic Acid	folic acid	Nature's Blend Folic Acid®, Folacin-800®	Needed in production of new red blood cells and helps anemia
Heart Stimulants	digoxin dobutamine dopamine epinephrine	Lanoxin®, Lanoxicaps®, Digitek® Dobutrex® Intropin® Adrenalin®	Makes heart beat stronger and slower

	inamrinone	Inocor®	
	isoproterenol	Isuprel®	
	metaraminol	Aramine®	
	milrinone	Primacor	
	norepinephrine	Levophed®	
	phenylephrine	Neo-Synephrine®	
Iron	ferrous gluconate	Fergon®	
	ferrous sulfate	Fer-in-Sol®, FeoSol®, Ferodan®, Slow-Fe®, Fero-Grad®	
	iron dextran	InFed®, DexFerrum®, Dexiron®, Infufer®	
	iron sucrose	Venofer®	
	sodium ferric gluconate complex	Ferrlecit®	
Male Hormone	fluoxymesterone	Halotestin®	Increase red blood cell production by stimulating bone marrow.
	methyltestosterone	Android®, Methitest®, Testred®, Virilon®	
	oxandrolone	Oxandrin®	

Vitamins	testosterone	Androderm®, Androgel®, Depo-Testosterone®	
	nandrolone	Deca-Durabolin®, Hybolin Decanoate®	
		Multi-vite®	Help maintain normal body functions and supplement vitamins in food.
		Nephro-Vite®	
		Nephro-vite + Fe®	
		Z-Bec®	
Vitamin D	calcitriol	Rocaltrol®, Calcijex®	Causes body to absorb calcium from food and place it in the bones.
	doxercalciferol	Hecterol®	
	ergocalciferol	Drisdol®	
	paricalcitol	Zemplar®	
Sleeping Pills and Tranquilizers	diazepam	Valium®, Diastat®	Aid in mental and physical relaxation; help to reduce insomnia, restlessness, itching and muscle cramps.
	secobarbital	Seconal®	
	phenobarbital	Luminal®	
	triazolam	Halcion®	
	temazepam	Restoril®	
	zolpidem tartrate	Ambien®	
	eszopiclone	Lunesta®	
	zaleplon	Sonata®	

ANTI-REJECTION MEDICATIONS

Calcineurin Inhibitors	cyclosporine	Neoral® Sandimmune® Generic: Gengraf®, Sidmak®, Eon®	Block T-cell activation and proliferation
	tacrolimus	Prograf®	
Corticosteroids	prednisone	Deltasone®	Stops antigen presentation and prevents the body from recognizing the transplanted kidney
Anti-proliferatives	azathioprine	Imuran®	Interferes with DNA and RNA synthesis so that T and B cell production is affected
	mycophenolate mofetil	Cellcept®	
	mycophenolate sodium	Myfortic®	
	sirolimus	Rapamune®	
	everolimus	Certican® - not yet FDA approved	

Notes

Internet Resources

American Association of Kidney Patients www.aakp.org	Information on patient education, conventions and newsletters to assist patients in being active participants in managing their disease. Download patient reference materials including Na-K Phos Counter and Protein/Calorie Counter.
Amgen www.lifeoptions.org	Order publications (mostly free) including rehabilitation information, & reproducible education sheets. "Showcase of Ideas" for patients and for professionals.
Amgen www.KidneySchool.org	20 minute learning modules on 16 different topics including nutrition, lab values, coping, staying active and alternative remedies. Pretest/posttest, graphics, pop-ups.
Baxter Healthcare www.renalinfo.com	Support and resources for people with kidney disease. Tips re lifestyle and travel, options for dialysis treatment, PD support, recipes, Patient of the Month, Kids Section and other resources. Includes information for different countries in different languages.
Cooking for David: A Culinary Dialysis Cookbook www.culinarykidneycooks.com	Weekly recipes, helpful hints and practical information for the dialysis diet. Can order *Cooking for David: A Culinary Dialysis Cookbook* through this website.
DaVita, Inc. www.davita.com	Tips, recipes, dialysis unit finder, interesting facts and articles
Davita Patient Citizens www.dialysispatients.org	DPC is an independent, nationwide, non-profit, patient-governed dialysis patient organization. Dedicated to improving dialysis patients' quality of life by developing awareness of dialysis-related issues, advocating for dialysis and pre-dialysis patients, improving the partnership between patients and caregivers, and promoting favorable public policy.
Hartwell Communication through grant from Watson Pharmaceuticals, Inc. www.iKidney.com	Nutrient charts, recipes, tips for patients and professionals. Includes Research library for renal related articles, renal dictionary, renal acronyms, nephrology pharmacy guide.
Renal Support Network www.renalnetwork.org	Education, advocacy, and employment site for kidney patients. RSN is a nationwide, non-profit, patient-governed kidney patient organization. Mission is to identify and meet the non-medical needs of those affected by chronic kidney disease. Founder and President Lori Hartwell.

Advance Directives

Ronald B. Miller, MD Clinical Professor of Medicine Emeritus, University of California, Irvine

Abstract or Summary of what will follow: Advance Directives: are also known as treatment directives (living wills or healthcare instruction directives) and proxy directives (durable powers of attorney for healthcare). These are instruments for planning in advance to ensure your values are respected and preferences honored even if you lose the ability to make healthcare decisions for yourself. However, before we discuss advance directives in detail, we should first consider medical decision-making both by patients able to make their own decisions and for patients who are unable to make decisions. And because modern medical technology allows life to be sustained that may be of such poor quality that patients may wish to limit treatment (if the treatment is burdensome or fails to achieve the patient's goals), we should also consider the patient's right to limit treatment before discussing advance directives.

Making medical decisions

> Patients and physicians need to answer several questions: The medical or scientific questions, "What is wrong?" and "What can be done about it?", and the ethical questions, "What should be done?" and "Who should decide?" In general the medical questions are answered by the doctor, the ethical questions by the patient.

In answering these questions it is helpful to keep in mind the goals of medicine:

- to maintain or restore health and prevent or cure illness
- to prevent suffering and relieve pain
- to reduce impairment and restore function
- to preserve the quality as well as the extent of life.

In addition, however, healthcare professionals need to know the goals and values of the individual patient. Health care professionals need to know the patient as a person (not simply the disease the patient has) and to know the patient's beliefs, values, attitudes, concerns, and preferences.

Given these general principles, all healthcare professionals may inform patients of their options, physicians recommend the options they believe best, and patients decide what to do (unless they have lost the ability to decide, in which case loved ones or appointed proxies can make decisions for them).

Medical Decision-Making:

Making decisions about interventions and treatments is a responsibility appropriately shared between doctor and patient.

"Decision-making capacity" and "decisional capacity" are medical terms for what in common language is called "competence" which technically is a legal term indicating decision-making capacity determined by a judge or court. Decision-making capacity is the ability to make decisions for yourself. It requires the ability to understand your illness, the expected consequences of the illness, and the nature, probable outcome, and possible risks of the proposed treatment, of alternative treatments, and of no treatment. The patient needs to be able to reason about the alternatives, to weigh the benefits and burdens of each, and to choose amongst them. Under the law, one is presumed competent until and unless determined otherwise in a court of law. Similarly, one is presumed to have decision-making capacity until and unless demonstrated to the contrary.

What is decision-making capacity (competence)?

What is informed decision-making (informed consent or refusal)? Informed consent or refusal is based upon the legal right to make healthcare decisions for yourself and to be provided the information necessary to do so. This right stems from the ethical principle of autonomy (self-rule) and the legal doctrine of self-determination (the right of individuals to determine what will be done to their own bodies). Informed consent or refusal, then, is decision-making about an intervention or treatment after having been informed of the nature and prognosis of one's illness, the treatment alternatives and their consequences and risks including those of no treatment, and after having the opportunity to ask questions in order to fully understand the options and their consequences.

What is required for informed consent or refusal? The information required for informed consent or refusal is the nature and prognosis of the illness, the benefits and risks of the recommended treatment and of alternative treatments, and the consequences of forgoing treatment. Obviously, you must have the capacity to understand this information and must be free of duress or coercion. In addition, you must be able to reason about the options and consequences, and also to communicate your decision. Although not mandatory, healthcare professionals are most appreciative if you are willing to communicate the reasons for your preference. This is particularly helpful in assessing your decision-making capacity though capacity should not be questioned simply because your decision is different from the decision that healthcare professionals would have made for themselves.

Are there constraints upon patient comprehension in informed consent? Patients are constrained in providing informed consent or refusal when they are given inadequate information, unexplained information, irrelevant information, distorted information, or even excessive information (information overload). Other factors that impair or preclude informed consent are the use of technical jargon by healthcare professionals, irrationality or immaturity of the patient, fear or other controlling influences, and coercion or manipulation by the healthcare professional or by the patient's family or friends (even when their intent is to help the patient).

Yes, there are three. In a true emergency (where failure to act would result in serious and imminent deterioration with risk to life, limb, sight, etc.) if one cannot communicate effectively with the patient or surrogate, the healthcare professional may proceed to treat the patient. Even in this circumstance it may be advisable to have documentation of the emergency and the recommended intervention by a second physician. A second exception is when the patient waives the right to informed consent, but under such circumstances the physician may wisely -- with permission, of course -- inform the patient's family of the patient's condition and recommended interventions or treatments. The third exception is in that rare circumstance that a person is a serious threat to him or herself or to others and in which the patient may legally be detained. Even then one may need court approval for treatment.

Are there exceptions to the requirement of informed consent or refusal?

Healthcare decisions should be expressed and discussed primarily in terms of the patient's goals. The goals, in turn, are based upon the patient's values and life experiences. Treatments are simply means to achieve goals, and even though they may have unpleasant or burdensome side effects which need to be understood by the patient, it is primarily the responsibility of the physician to recommend treatment based upon the patient's goals and preferences.

Why should one emphasize goals, not treatments?

Although it may be unpleasant, even frightening, to contemplate and discuss serious and particularly lethal illness, it is important to do so in order to plan for the future we will all face sooner or later. It is particularly important important to do so in advance when we are still competent, in order to plan for the possibility that

How can one discuss and plan for serious, and particularly terminal, illness?

we could become unable to understand our illness or to make decisions about its treatment. And it is important even if we are in good health and do not have a familial or occupational predisposition to predictable and identifiable illness or injury. This may then require speculation about a variety of possible illnesses or injuries and the varied courses they might follow or complications that might develop. If one already has a condition such as progressive kidney dysfunction, the course and possible complications may be predictable and allow more specific planning. In any event, one should contemplate and discuss future possibilities with one's family and appointed surrogate (agent) and particularly with one's physician.

How important is my choice of physician, and what qualities should I look for?

Extremely important: Besides your illness and your own preferences and goals, the most important factors determining your health care and satisfaction with it are your physician and his or her competence and qualities. Everyone should have a primary care physician with a long-standing, compassionate and empathetic relationship of mutual respect and care. Primary care is best provided by an internist, family physician, or geriatrician except in the case of children for whom a pediatrician is appropriate and in the case of some otherwise healthy young women for whom an obstetrician-gynecologist may be appropriate. For patients with specific serious and chronic conditions an internist with subspecialty training (e.g., a nephrologist for patients with kidney failure) may be the best and most efficient provider of primary care. It is extremely important that your primary care physician know your life history, family values, religious or spiritual beliefs, personal goals, and what you hope to accomplish. He or she should have leadership qualities: be an effective quarterback with consulting physicians and be willing to coordinate and direct your care and to make the difficult decisions with and for you. He or she should be nonjudgmental and conscious of his or her own values but willing to act upon your values and goals and truly open to shared decision-making. He or she should be an open-minded and effective communicator willing to listen and to take the time necessary, even allowing time for you to adjust to bad news. These characteristics are important for your family as well as for you, the patient. Because you may have serious events in the course of your illness, the ideal physician should be comfortable in the intensive care unit, but also skilled in palliative care with willingness to treat symtoms appropriately. And when the time comes, your physician should understand your end-of-life preferences and be willing to advocate for you.

Limiting Treatment:

You may find illness unbearable or that the burdens of treatment exceed the benefits.

Yes, you may. Although the decision had precedential authority only in New Jersey, the Supreme Court of that state in the celebrated case of Karen Ann Quinlan held that mechanical ventilation could be discontinued at the request of her parents because there was no chance of her returning to a cognitive and sapient state. Even though discontinuation of the ventilator did not result in her death as had been expected, her parents did not request removal of the feeding tube which allowed her to survive nine years in an unconscious state. Somewhat more than a decade later, the US Supreme Court in the case of Nancy Beth Cruzan (a young Missouri woman who was permanently unconscious following an automobile accident) held that there is a constitutional right to refuse treatment, including artificial nutrition and hydration, and that this right is not lost if a person becomes incompetent (in which case the right may be exercised by a surrogate), and this right does not require that one have a terminal

May I refuse treatment, even life-sustaining treatment?

condition. However, the Court held that the State could require clear and convincing evidence of a patient's wishes, and this has had the beneficial outcome that many people now execute advance directives.

Why might I forgo life-sustaining treatment?

You might request that life-sustaining treatment be discontinued because it failed to restore you to a state satisfactory to you. This might be due to the severity of the illness for which you were receiving the life-sustaining treatment, but it might also be due to a different or antecedent or subsequent illness and disability. You might also decide to discontinue life-sustaining treatment because the treatment itself was so burdensome. Many, but by no means all, individuals who are permanently ventilator dependent prefer not to continue to live on mechanical ventilation indefinitely. Some individuals even find the burdens of kidney failure and of dialysis to outweigh the benefits.

Might such a preference be misunderstood or ignored?

Yes, a request to forgo or to discontinue life-sustaining treatment might be considered suicidal and irrational. And if thought irrational or suicidal, a physician might ignore the request. This should, of course, initiate discussions which would allow the physician to evaluate the decisional capacity of the patient and the rationale of the request. Not infrequently a psychiatrist might be consulted to further evaluate decisional capacity, and if it was thought that the patient were a danger to him or herself, the patient might be legally detained and, with court permission, treated.

Is there a difference between withdrawing and withholding treatment?

Yes, and no. For most patients, families, and physicians it is emotionally more difficult to withdraw than to withhold treatment. On the other hand, it is usually held that there is no ethical or legal difference. Although this is true in general, under certain circumstances there may be a difference. For example, if a patient is unaware that a treatment for his or her condition is available, and if the patient would benefit from that treatment (benefit in the judgment of the patient, not others), it would be unethical to withhold the treatment. The rub, of course, is that the physician might believe the patient would not benefit and would simply suffer undergoing the treatment (if the patient chose to start the treament in the mistaken belief it would be helpful), and thus the physician might believe it was unethical to recommend the treatment or even, perhaps, to inform the patient of the existence of such treatment. Wherever there is uncertainty about the benefits (or the burdens) of a treatment, it is appropriate to inform the patient of the treatment, and it may be appropriate for the patient to undergo a trial of treatment. The shared decision might be for the trial to be time-limited with criteria for adequate success or excessive burdens to be determined and agreed upon in advance.

What is CPR?

CPR stands for Cardiopulmonary Resuscitation. It is a coordinated set of treatments for the purpose of reestablishing cardiac (heart) and pulmonary (lung) function when either the heart stops beating or the lungs stop breathing or both. CPR consists of breathing for the patient (usually via a mask or a tube in the windpipe) and of manually compressing the chest to "massage" the heart to pump blood throughout the body. Oxygen and medications are usually given, and if the electrical activity of the heart is deranged (e.g., ventricular fibrillation), electric shock may be delivered to the heart by electrodes applied to the chest wall in an effort to restore a normal heart rhythm and beat. The purpose, of course, is to prevent death and, by prompt initiation of CPR, to prevent brain damage.

Can I refuse CPR? And why might I wish to do so?

When a person has cardiac and/or pulmonary arrest, she/he promptly loses consciousness and becomes unable either to consent to, or to refuse, CPR. However, some individuals who are terminally and burdensomely ill or who simply suffer physically and/or emotionally may wish that CPR not be attempted should they have a cardiac and/or pulmonary arrest. They may so request.

What is a DNR or DNAR request or order?

Increasingly health professionals prefer the term "DNAR" (meaning "do not attempt resuscitation") to the term "DNR" (meaning "do not resuscitate") because unlike the high rate of success of cardiopulmonary resuscitation on the television show, "ER", the success of CPR, even for patients observed in the hospital, is significantly less than 10%. A Do-Not-Attempt Resuscitation (DNAR) request is a request of a patient (or if the patient is decisionally incapacitated, a request of the surrogate decision-maker) that CPR not be undertaken if there is a cardiac and/ or pulmonary arrest. A DNAR order is the written order of the physician not to provide CPR if there is a cardiac and/or pulmonary arrest. The purpose of the order is to inform all health care professionals in the hospital or nursing home not to initiate cardiopulmonary resuscitation in the event of an arrest. Most often this is an order written in the hospital or nursing home chart of a patient, almost always at the request of the patient or surrogate (though the recommendation may be initiated by the physician if he or she believes the patient unlikely to benefit from CPR). However, in some jurisdictions an out-of-hospital DNAR is allowed by law if the patient or surrogate and physician sign an appropriate form (and in some jurisdictions where a necklace pendant or a bracelet inscribed "DNAR" is worn by the patient).

Since I can refuse treatment, can I demand it?

Certainly you can request treatment, and even demand it, but you may not always receive it. You may request treatment even if it was not recommended or offered by your physician, and if the request is reasonable, surely it will be provided. A conflict may occur, however, if you or your family believe the request appropriate, but the physician and/or his consultants do not. A physician's professional medical ethic (to do good, to do no harm, and to allow patients to choose from among effective, beneficial treatments) does not entitle a patient to non-beneficial, ineffective, inappropriate, or harmful treatment. A conflict arises if you judge the requested treatment to be appropriate, but the physician does not.

What if the doctor and I (or my family) disagree?

Fortunately, in the overwhelming majority of decisions to be made in health care, physicians and patients agree. Occasionally, however, there are different opinions about what you need, about the goals of treatment, about the probability of benefit from, or efficacy of, the treatment, and occasionally these differences are based upon different moral beliefs, and rarely upon different judgements whether a treatment is "worth it". Most differences resolve with discussion or with negotiation and compromise, and occasionally with new insights provided by consultation with other healthcare professionals or with an ethics committee. When differences become intractable disputes, resolution may require mediation, transfer to another physician or institution or — as a last resort — adjudication by a judge in court.

Can a doctor or institution refuse to provide treatment?

Yes, of course, doctors and institutions may refuse to provide treatment, and in some jurisdictions this may be legal. For example, California law permits physicians or institutions to refuse interventions or treatments on the basis of conscience or of ineffectiveness of the intervention or treatment. However, the law does require a reasonable effort to transfer the patient if the patent or family believes the treatment or intervention should be provided. In Texas the patient or surrogate is given 48 hours to participate in an ethics or medical committee review, and if the review finds the treatment inappropriate, the treatment may be withdrawn after it is continued for 10 days to allow for an opportunity to transfer the patient. Patients or families, of course, may go to court hoping for an injunction against the withdrawal of treatment.

Decision-Making for Those Who Lack Decision-Making Capacity:

What is a lack of decision-making capacity (decisional incapacity) and how does it differ from incompetence?

A lack of decision-making capacity is the inability to make decisions (or to give informed consent or refusal). The inability may be global, invariable, and persistent or it may be partial, variable, and temporary. It may be due to a loss of consciousnesss or to an inability to understand, to reason, or to express oneself. In common discourse we might call decisional incapacity "incompetence." However, "competence" is a legal term. Under the law one is presumed competent unless one is a minor or until one has been declared incompetent in a court of law.

What are the criteria for incapacity (incompetence)?

As does the law, we should presume an individual or patient has decisional capacity until we have evidence otherwise. The criteria for incapacity are a lack of recognition of one's condition and its seriousness, an inability to understand information one is provided and its significance, an inability to reason and process the information, to understand the benefits and risks of an intervention or treatment and of alternative interventions or treatments, or to make and to communicate a decision. Capacity is, however, specific to the decision that must be made. One might be able to state that one wishes his or her spouse to make complex healthcare decisions yet be unable to make those decisions oneself. Although one would hope that decisions were reasoned, they need not be reasonable. Although an unreasonable decision by a patient may lead the healthcare professional to suspect incapacity, it is not sufficient to judge incapacity since individuals have the right to idiosyncratic beliefs, preferences, and choices.

How can decisions be made for patients who lack capacity?

In the past, physicians paternalistically (since many physicians now are women we could say maternalistically or parentalistically) often made unilateral decisions regarding the care of patients who lacked capacity. They prescribed what — in their judgment — was in the best interest of the patient. Advanced medical technology, however, now allows many treatments that not all patients would want. Furthermore, we now believe that patients have the right to be informed and to make decisions for themselves. We no longer accept the notion that a health-care professional may speak on behalf of the patient without capacity. Rather, we insist on a proxy or surrogate decision-maker to either consent or refuse recommendations that are made by the physician.

The standards for decision making and for providing information (for the patient's informed consent or refusal) have evolved from what the reasonable physician or professional would decide or provide, to what the reasonable patient would decide or wish to know, to what the particular patient would decide or would find material to his or her decision.

The answers to subsequent questions regarding proxies, surrogates, agents, and attorneys-in-fact apply not simply to decision-making for patients who lack capacity, but also to specific legally-authorized decision making for individuals who have executed an advance directive and have become incompetent.

What is a proxy, a surrogate decision-maker, or agent?

A proxy (literally a person who cares for another's interests) or surrogate (literally one who is asked for, or who is a substitute) is a person authorized or appointed to act for another. Generally, the two words ("proxy" and "surrogate") may be used interchangeably, though in some jurisdictions they are defined differently in the law. An agent also is one authorized to act for another, but we rarely use the word unless the agent is so authorized by legislation or adjudication. In all states one may appoint a proxy to make healthcare decisions if the principal loses decision-making capacity. In some states the individual who may legally serve as a proxy or surrogate is defined by statutory law, in others by common-law (that is, by the precedent of court-decided cases).

What is an agent, agent-in-fact or attorney-in-fact? An agent, agent-in-fact, or attorney-in-fact is an individual appointed in a power of attorney or a durable power of attorney to act for another.

Who is the legal proxy? Commonly, the proxy or surrogate with legal priority or highest standing is either an attorney-in-fact appointed by the principal in a durable power-of-attorney, or is a conservator or guardian appointed by a court. Next is a spouse (and in some jurisdictions a domestic partner), followed by a parent or adult child and, and then by a sibling. Only thereafter come more distant relatives, caretakers, or friends. Under emergency circumstances, however, in most jurisdictions a physician (or two physicians) may make decisions without approval of a surrogate.

Who is the morally-valid proxy? The morally valid surrogate or proxy is an individual who has significant involvement with the principal, knowledge of his or her values, willingness to express those values or wishes, and no emotional or other conflict of interest that would interfere with making appropriate decisions for the individual. The morally valid proxy may in some jurisdictions be lower in the hierarchy than the legally valid proxy, and if the two have different understandings of what the patient would wish or what is in the patient's best interests, there is a serious ethical problem. Unless the legal proxy would defer to the morally valid proxy, the healthcare provider (physician or institution) might wish to take the issue to court.

What are the characteristics of an ideal surrogate or proxy (agent)? A good proxy should know you and know (or be willing to learn) your values, beliefs, concerns, preferences, and goals. He or she should be available, able, and willing to speak for you and to advocate your values and choices. Additionally, he or she should be willing to meet with you and your physician in order to learn about your health, your condition, your prognosis, and what might be expected in terms of the course and complications of your illness or illnesses. The ideal proxy is trustworthy, articulate, responsible, persistent, and assertive (though diplomatic), and would be able and willing to confront anyone who challenges your choices or attempts to interfere with achieving your goals and treatment preferences. A good proxy understands the healthcare and legal systems or is sufficiently resourceful to learn whatever is needed in order to effect your wishes — if necessary, through consultants, an ethics committee, or even an attorney or court.

For a patient who lacks decisional capacity, the doctor recommends and the proxy decides. It is very important that the proxy states not what he or she would personally want, but rather what you, the patient, would want. Whenever possible a proxy should make decisions based upon your (the principal's) express wishes. Ideally you and your proxy together with your physician will have discussed your illness, its likely course, and all foreseeable complications such that you have had an opportunity to state explicitly what you would wish under various circumstances. When circumstances arise that could not have been predicted or that you failed to consider in advance, decisions should be based upon substituted judgment. That is, your proxy should judge what you would wish, based upon his or her knowledge of your values, your goals, and what you might have said about someone with a similar problem. Only when this is not possible should the decision be based upon a judgment of what is in your best interest (from your perspective). Even that can take into account matters that you might feel relevant such as the welfare of your loved ones, and even your financial preferences (e.g., if you would prefer to finance your grandchild's college education rather than dissipating your savings on your own terminal illness). This example, is actually substituted judgment rather than an isolated best interest judgment most of which

How do, and how should, proxies (surrogates) make decisions for patients who lack capacity?

are, as in the California law, to be made considering "the principal's personal values to the extent known to the agent". Unfortunately, substituted judgments and best interest judgments are not perfect. Proxies, especially if loved ones, sometimes overestimate, at other times underestimate, what treatment the patient would want. Nevertheless, in the absence of clear treatment directives or express wishes, proxy judgments are the best we have (and may be somewhat closer to what patients would want than are judgments by physicians).

What should my proxy know in deciding whether or not to be my agent?

In deciding whether or not to be your agent, an individual you might ask to be, should know you and your goals and values well enough to decide whether he or she is comfortable advocating your goals and values for you. For example, if the circumstance were one in which you would wish life-sustaining treatment discontinued, would your proxy be emotionally capable of so requesting. He or she might also wish to consider the time, effort, as well as the emotional stamina required to advocate for you. In addition, he or she might wish to meet your primary physician in order to know whether they could reasonably negotiate if the physician's preferences and recommendations were different from yours.

How much authority will my agent have?

Unless you limit the authority of the agent, in most jurisdictions your agent would have the same authority as you.

What should I do if there is no one I trust to be my proxy?

If there is no one you trust to be your proxy, since a proxy is not mandatory, you may wish to have a treatment or healthcare directive without a proxy directive. If that is the case, you should expect to expend significant time and energy consulting with your physician about your health, possible illnesses and their courses and complications in order to reasonably consider what you would want and not want under all likely circumstances. You would also wish to articulate your values and your goals so that if you developed conditions or complications that you have not anticipated, others could reasonably judge what you would want. Particularly important would be considering what circumstances would be worse than death such that you would prefer not to receive treatment of life-threatening illness or would prefer that food and fluid (or medically administered nutrition and hydration) be withheld so that you might die in a few days or at most a few weeks.

Another option is to seek a professional proxy. A health-care professional whom you know but who is not directly involved in your care and yet who is willing to serve in this capacity could be a good choice. Alternatively, you may wish to consult one or more of the resources listed at the end of this chapter.

> **Advance Directives:** *Planning in advance to ensure your values are respected and preferences honored even if you lose the ability to make healthcare decisions for yourself.*

An advance directive (that is, a directive made in advance of decisional incapacity, not an "advanced" directive) is either a health care or treatment directive (specifying what one would or would not want under various circumstances) or a proxy directive (naming the individual, and preferably alternate individuals, that one would wish to make decisions if one were unable to make decisions for him or herself), or both a treatment and a proxy directive. The latter, that is the directive that both specifies treatment and names one or more proxies, is called a combined advance directive. Ideally advance directives should be written documents signed and dated not only by the principal but also by witnesses and/or by a notary (and if the patient is in a nursing home, also by an ombudsperson). In California if the document is unavailable at the time of hospitalization

What is an advance directive, a combined advance directive?

(or if there is no document) health care personnel can ask the patient to name proxies and to state treatment preferences, and if these are documented in the chart they serve as a legal advance directive (until the advance directive document is brought into the hospital, or for the duration of the hospitalization, or 60 days, whichever is shorter).

What is a proxy directive? A proxy directive names an individual or individuals to make decisions on behalf of the principal. It is generally thought best to name a single individual rather than multiple individuals to make decisions, but it is also wise to name alternates in a preferred sequence to be consulted if the first named individual is unavailable. There are, however, cultures that prefer decisions to be made by the entire family rather than by a single individual, and the physician should take this into consideration even though not required by law. Normally a proxy does not make decisions for the principal until the principal has become unable to make decisions for him or herself. However, California law allows the principal to indicate that decisional authority is granted the proxy immediately (if so desired by the principal), even though the principal is still decisionally capable.

What is a treatment directive? A treatment or healthcare directive, often called a "living will", is a statement or statements of treatment preferences ideally related to the patient's goals and values. Most commonly the statements limit treatment under certain conditions, and historically treatment limitation documents were called "living wills". However, one may also request treatment, even treatment that others might not wish, but physicians and hospitals need not legally provide such treatment if it is illegal (for example, physician-assisted suicide except in Oregon or euthanasia in all states) and, in California, if it is against the conscience of the physician or against a policy of conscience of the hospital or if the treatment would be ineffective. When legal treatment is not to be provided, reasonable efforts to transfer the patient to a willing provider are required by law. As previously noted, legislation with similar intent to avoid what is often called "futile treatment" has been enacted in Texas.

How are advance directives useful?

Ideally an advance directive allows for decisions to be made for a patient who has lost the ability to make decisions for him or herself precisely as the patient would wish them made were he or she still able to make decisions. This, of course, is the intent but unfortunately not always the reality. Nevertheless, the uncertainty for both physicians and for family members who, in the absence of an advance directive, must make decisions for a patient without reasonable knowledge of what the patient would want is largely avoided by advance proxy and/or treatment directives. Even when the patient's preferences are not known from explicit expressed wishes and cannot reasonably be inferred (substituted judgment) from the patient's known values, a proxy directive allows for legal decision making and avoids the delays and inefficiency of having to go to court.

Do I need both a proxy directive and a treatment directive?

Ideally yes, legally no. Most health-care professionals strongly advise a proxy directive except for the very rare patient who has no one he or she wishes or trusts to make decisions for him or her after the loss of decisional capacity. And a proxy directive alone is sufficient if the proxy knows the patient thoroughly and would make decisions precisely as the patient would or if the principal prefers the proxy's judgment to his or her own (for example, if the principal wishes the proxy to make decisions based on the welfare of the principal's family, not the welfare of the principal alone). A proxy directive alone is also sufficient if the patient has provided (on or off the record) sufficient information upon which treatment decisions can be made reliably. Most would think the optimal way of doing so would be to have a treatment as well as a proxy directive even though it is rare that one can express treatment preferences for all circumstances that might befall him or her. Ideally, then, both proxy and treatment directives are useful and complement each other, but legally one need not have both, and legally one can have either or both, or neither.

What is the purpose of an advance directive? From the perspective of the principal, advance directives are intended to ensure that the principal's values and dignity are honored and preferences are followed. From the standpoint of the principal's family advance directives ideally provide comfort in knowing what the patient would want under various circumstances. From the standpoint of the physician and the hospital or nursing home, advance directives allow for reasonably efficient decision-making and avoid the liability of not going to court or the delay and inefficiency of going to court for direction.

What are the consequences of not having an advance directive? Not having an advance directive for health care risks healthcare decisions that are not of one's preference and thus potentially not in one's best interests taking into account one's values and preferences. In addition, not having an advance directive is a disservice to one's loved ones and one's physician and hospital since, even if it does not result in significant delays and inefficiencies of care, it does not provide the comfort to one's family and physician of knowing they are acting as you would wish them to.

Is a DNAR request an advance directive? Yes and no. Conceptually a DNAR request is an advance treatment directive (refusal of CPR). In practice, however, a request for a DNAR order is not usually thought of as an advance directive. One reason is that all other treatment and proxy directives are durable; that is, they become operative if the patient loses decisional capacity, and they last permanently (or for a number of years, as specified in the statutes of various states). In contrast, a DNAR order in a hospital lasts only for the specific hospitalization or stay in a long-term-care facility, and must be rewritten for each admission if the patient and physician want it to continue. Many hospitals have policies that require the DNAR order to be reviewed more frequently, and of course they should be reviewed if there is improvement in the patient's clinical condition. Until recently, patients rarely mentioned cardiopulmonary resuscitation in advance treatment directives, but when this is done a request for CPR or a request not to attempt resuscitation would be a legal advance directive just as is any other request for treatment or treatment omission.

If an individual's health or life circumstances change significantly, a DNAR request or order should be reconsidered, and either reaffirmed or suspended. This is true for all treatment directives: Ideally they should be reviewed periodically, and as a practical matter they should be reviewed whenever the health or life circumstances of the individual changes.

Should DNAR orders and advanced directives be reviewed?

POLST stands for physician orders for life sustaining treatment, POST for physician orders for scope of treatment, and MOLST for medical orders for life sustaining treatment. These are physician orders, not a patient's or individual's advance directive though clearly the physician considers the patient's preferences in writing these orders. Unlike orders in a hospital, however, these orders are intended to direct the care of the patient not only in the hospital, but in a nursing home or wherever the patient may reside. The concept was developed in Oregon and has been adopted in a number of jurisdictions: e.g., POLST in Oregon, Washington, and Utah, POST in West Virginia and MOLST in Rochester, New York. The PIT is a form for physician documentation of preferred intensity of treatment developed by the California Medical Association for use in long-term care facilities. The Council on Ethical Affairs of the CMA considered its possible use

What is a POLST, POST, MOLST or PIT?

in care settings other than nursing homes.

POLST is a standardized order sheet with alternative orders in several categories reflecting the patent's preferences for provision or omission of intensive treatment, cardiopulmonary resuscitation, antibiotics, and nutrition and hydration. The POLST order form is printed on brightly colored paper so that it and be easily located in an emergency, and when enabled by state law it is applicable if the patent is in a nursing home, hospice, or at home as well as in the hospital. Perhaps the most important benefit is that it requires discussion by the physician with the patient and/or surrogate, and it converts patent's preferences (which are often vague or irrelevant to the circumstances that befall the patient) into medically appropriate and understandable action items. Thus, POLST increases the likelihood of a patient's preferences being followed, and it is a valuable supplement to the patient's advance directive. For additional information see www.polst.org.

What is a living will? A living will is a treatment directive, usually a treatment-limitation directive. In the narrow sense, it is a brief, often generic or standardized statement, such as the following: "If the situation should arise in which there is no reasonable expectation that I will recover from an incapacitating physical disability or mental infirmity, I request that I be allowed to die and not be kept alive by artificial means or heroic measures." In the broad sense, a living will is any statement (commonly written rather than oral) by a competent individual regarding his or her preference for treatment, or treatment limitation, or regarding who should make such decisions should the individual become incapacitated. It is called a "living will" because, unlike a normal testamentary or property will which becomes effective only after death, a living will becomes effective during one's life, though usually only after one has become unable to speak capably for him or herself. The generic or standardized statement provided above as an example of a living will is a poor example of a treatment directive because it is vague and thus subject to variable interpretation. Although the individual making such a statement might have a clear idea of what he or she meant by "artificial means or heroic measures", these words mean different things to different individuals. This could also be said of "incapacitating physical disability or mental infirmity" and of "a reasonable expectation of recovery". Thus, despite an understanding that the individual would not want "everything done that could be done", the physician or proxy might have great difficulty knowing what treatments to provide and what to omit under a variety of circumstances.

What is a "good" advance directive?

There is diversity of opinion regarding this question, and a good advance directive for one individual may be different from a good directive for another. Some believe one should have only a proxy directive and not a treatment directive because it is so difficult to imagine which of the many potential complications of even a known specific illness one may develop. Others believe treatment directives are helpful so long as they are general enough to guide a physician and proxy, but not so specific as to constrain or restrict their making decisions for you that you might make differently than stated in the advance directive because of unexpected complications of the illness or its treatment, different coexistent conditions, or changes in the context that you could not have predicted. Still others believe treatment directives should be as specific as possible stating not only your goals for treatment, but also your values, where you would wish to be treated, and specific preferences for treatment in a variety of specific — albeit hypothetical — circumstances.

Generally a good advance directive is a combined advance directive naming a proxy and alternate or successor proxies and stating treatment preferences or declinations. An advance treatment directive should be clinically applicable and sensible, clear and understandable, reliable and reproducible, valid and effective with documentation of the individual's goals and rationale. It should indicate whether it is to be interpreted literally or with leeway permitting the proxy or physician or both to override if they believe what the patient stated would no longer be in his or her best interest. Indeed, whether some flexibility and exceptions are permitted, certainly individuals should revise their advance directive if their condition or circumstances change.

How general or how specific should a treatment directive be? A treatment directive should be general enough to apply to unanticipated circumstances, yet specific enough to offer clear guidance. In an article entitled, "Enough: the failure of the living will" (Hastings Center Report 34 (2): 30-42, 2004), Fagerlin and Schneider stated in order to guide treatment, living wills tended to be too general, but "the demand for specificity forced patients to address more questions than they could comprehend. So, generalities were insufficiently specific and insufficiently considered. Specifics were insufficiently general and perhaps still insufficiently considered." Let me, however, give some examples of both general and specific treatment directives.

General treatment directives:

Answers to the following questions provide general guidance:

What provides pleasure and gives meaning in your life?

What physical condition would you find intolerable?

What mental incapacity would you find intolerable?

What are minimally acceptable physical and mental capacities?

Are there religious or philosophic tenets so important that they should guide medical decisions for you?

Can you tell us what you would want and what you would not want were you in a condition similar to that of Karen Ann Quinlan, Nancy Beth Cruzan, Theresa Marie Schiavo, or Robert Wendland?

Specific advance directives:

Answers to the following questions provide more specific guidance:

If you should lose the ability to make healthcare decisions for yourself, whom do you wish to appoint to make decisions with your physician?

Is there a physician you would prefer if life and death decisions had to be made?

How much leeway should your proxy and/or physician have to override your stated treatment preferences if they believed those preferences were no longer in your best interest (e.g., if a new treatment for your condition became available)?

Are there circumstances in which you would wish your suffering and life to end?

Are there circumstances in which you would wish to not begin or to discontinue dialysis?

Are there circumstances in which you would prefer life-sustaining treatment (such as dialysis) to be discontinued?

If you were not dependent upon life-sustaining treatment, are there circumstances in which you would wish to forgo food and fluid (whether by mouth or by feeding tube or intravenous administration) in order to hasten your dying?

What is a power of attorney?
A power of attorney is a written appointment of another individual as the principal's agent to perform specific acts or kinds of acts, commonly legal, financial, or personal. The power may be general or limited and lasts only during the life of the principal. A durable power-of-attorney remains effective even if the principal is disabled.

What is a durable power-of-attorney for healthcare (DPAHC)?
A durable power of attorney for healthcare is a written document that appoints another individual (or successor individuals) as proxy to make healthcare decisions on behalf of the principal, usually only after the principal loses the ability to make decisions for him or herself. It is durable not only in continuing despite loss of decisional capacity by the principal but also in remaining valid indefinitely (or at least for a number of years) and valid in allowing post-mortem decisions such as autopsy, disposition of organs, burial or cremation, and funeral or memorial service if not otherwise arranged. Many believe this proxy directive is the best type of advance directive because it allows you to appoint almost any adult in whom you have great confidence to make decisions for you in the future under circumstances that can rarely be foreseen with sufficient certainty to allow you to make those decisions clearly and specifically in advance. The first durable power of attorney for healthcare legislation was enacted in California and became effective in 1984.

What was the Natural Death Act?
The California Natural Death Act (1976) was the first statutory advance directive. It allowed individuals to direct that their physician withhold or withdraw life-sustaining treatment in the event of terminal illness or permanent

unconsciousness, and it provided immunity to a physician or hospital who withheld or withdrew life-sustaining treatment. The act has been superseded in California by the Health Care Decisions Law of 2000.

Are advance directives legal documents?

Yes, all states have treatment directives (living wills) and/or proxy directives (durable powers of attorney for healthcare). Laws vary from state to state, however, and for an advance directive to be legal it should conform to the requirements of the state in which it is to be relied upon. Since the overwhelming majority of physicians and hospitals respect the rights of patients to name a proxy or to forgo treatment when it is viewed as more burdensome than beneficial, the legality of advance directives should be more a technicality than a necessity. However, technical compliance with the law has proven to be of extreme importance in a number of states and in various circumstances. Several states require clear and convincing evidence (as did Missouri in the case of Nancy Beth Cruzan, a requirement upheld by the US Supreme Court) of the patient's preferences to withhold or withdraw life-sustaining treatment. Additional states require specific evidence of the patient's preferences if life-sustaining treatment is to be withheld or withdrawn (a) unless the patient is in a terminal condition or a state of permanent unconsciousness (as in the Robert Wendland case in California) or (b) if nutrition and hydration are to be omitted (existing or pending legislation in several states following the Theresa Marie Schiavo case in Florida).

Are copies of advance directives legal?

In most, if not all, states copies of that state's advance directives (or of the advance directives of other states that essentially comply with the specific state's requirements) are considered legal. However, advance directives are automatically rescinded if a new advance directive is written, and one might not appreciate that an advance directive copy had been superseded. Thus, it is wise to keep a list of the numbers of copies made and to whom they have been entrusted so that outdated copies can be recovered and either destroyed or lined through and labeled rescinded with the date and a signature. I prefer the latter, rather than destruction of outdated originals and copies since questions may arise with regard to whether or not an advance directive was rescinded and whether a physician had acted in compliance with an advance directive.

Are advance directives legal in other states? A single advance directive form, that of "Five Wishes" (the form of the organization, Aging with Dignity -- see Resources at the end of this chapter) is said to be legal in 37 states. California has a model advance directive in its statute, but does not require that that specific form be used, and allows directives from other states that essentially comply with California law to be honored in California. Your doctor or a social worker in your dialysis unit or renal center should be able to advise you where to obtain forms, and may be very helpful in discussing your particular circumstances and the advisability of executing an advance directive. Witnessing by a notary or other appropriate witness or witnesses is necessary for written directives to be legal.

Do I need an attorney to draw up an advance directive? No, though some individuals prefer to have an attorney draft their advance directives or at least advise them in doing so. An attorney's statement might be required, however, if one wished to include in his or her advance directive a statement prohibiting specific individuals from petitioning the court to challenge the individual's advance directive.

How should I discuss my wishes with my proxy and with my physician? Thoroughly and repeatedly: It is important not only that your proxy and your physician know your preferences and goals for treatment, but also that you understand thoroughly what you intend and why. It is also important that your physician advise you if he or she believes what you have stated you wish is not in your best interest (perhaps because you have misunderstood your condition or the treatment and its benefits and burdens). It is optimal to meet with your proxy and physician together and have a three-way conversation about your condition, its treatment, your preferences and goals.

Although certainly not necessary, it could prove important in honoring your preferences to have documentation of your proxy's and physician's understanding of your preferences and of their willingness to comply with those preferences.

Should I get my proxy and my physician to sign acceptance of my advance directive?

The Patient Self-Determination Act is a federal statute requiring hospitals, long-term care facilities, hospice programs, home health agencies, and prepaid health plans (HMO's) to provide information upon admission concerning one's rights under state law to accept or refuse treatment and to formulate advance directives, and also information concerning the policies of the provider or organization respecting the implementation of such rights. They must also comply with state law respecting advance directives, document whether a patient has or does not have an advance directive, and educate hospital staff and community on issues concerning advance directives. Unfortunately the time of admission to a hospital, nursing home, hospice, or dialysis facility is not an ideal time for patients to consider all of the circumstances and issues basic to formulating an advance directive. Not only is the admission usually emotionally upsetting, but thinking through what one would want or not want under a variety of serious circumstances – as required to formulate a treatment directive – is itself emotionally challenging. Thus, now is the best time to formulate an advance directive.

What is the Patient Self-Determination Act (PSDA)?

The Patient Self-Determination Act did not include dialysis units amongst the institutions required to provide information and document whether or not you have an advance directive. However, recently the ESRD (End Stage Renal Disease) Workgroup of Promoting Excellence in End-of-Life Care (a national program office of the Robert Wood Johnson Foundation) recommended to the CMS (Centers for Medicare and Medicaid Services) that the "Conditions of Participation" for dialysis units "include requirements for advance care planning and the provision of palliative care." If you have an advance directive you should present a copy at the time of admission to a dialysis facility. If you do not already have an advance directive, since the initiation of dialysis is overwhelming for most individuals, the National Kidney Foundation recommends that unless you indicate a desire for further discussion at the time of admission, you should be provided information within a month of initiation of dialysis. And if you do not wish to discuss or execute an advance directive at that time, the National Kidney Foundation suggests you be approached again within three months by which time most patients have "reached a level of comfort with dialysis and with the staff."

What is the benefit of having an advance directive? Probably the greatest benefit of drafting an advance directive is having thought about your health and illness and treatment options in relation to your values, goals, and preferences. Thus, if you are suddenly faced with making medical decisions you are better prepared to do so. In addition, drafting an advance directive should trigger discussions with your physician and with your family and friends. Even if a legal document is not completed or preferences are not written out, such discussions go a long way to protect your right to receive or to refuse treatment should you lose the ability to speak for yourself. Furthermore, it greatly reduces the burden on your family and your physician who would have to make decisions for you if you became too ill to do so for yourself and too ill to know your treatment preferences and whom you might wish to make decisions for you. It also provides the physician and the proxy with legal protection when they follow your wishes.

Are there disadvantages of having an advance directive?

Although, in the vast majority of instances the advantages greatly outweigh the disadvantages, there can be disadvantages of having an advance directive. Sometimes professionals, relatives, or friends who only know that you have one, jump to the conclusion that you would not want life-sustaining treatment. This might be true even if your directive actually indicated you would want such treatment or even if the directive simply named whom you want to make decisions for you. Another potential disadvantage is that you might fail to update the advance directive when you changed your mind concerning either treatment or proxy preferences. Yet another disadvantage is likely if your treatment directive is poorly or vaguely written and is inadequately clarified in discussions with your physician and proxy. Indeed, discussion is probably the most important benefit of executing an advance directive. Discussion helps to clarify your own understanding of your illness as well as to clarify and articulate your beliefs, values, and preferences -- particularly those that influence decisions about your health care. In turn, this helps you communicate your wishes clearly to your physician, proxy, and loved ones.

What is a values history?

A values history is an inventory of answers to questions about your living environment, your family and friends, your religious background and beliefs, your attitudes toward life in general and toward independence and control, health, doctors, illness, death and dying, and finances. The values history may ask whether you have preferences regarding specific medical procedures (such as dialysis, transplantation, mechanical ventilation, medically-administered nutrition and hydration, organ donation) and whether you have any written documents, particularly advance directives. It might also ask your preferences regarding autopsy, burial or cremation, funeral, eulogy, and obituary. When such questions were developed for public guardians to ask friends of solitary, incapacitated patients what the patients believed or had said about their beliefs, values, health and treatment preferences in order to guide the guardian to make appropriate decisions for individuals without decisional capacity or surrogate, it became evident that such questions could be helpful to anyone to clarify his or her own values and to articulate them and, preferably to record them for use by a surrogate should he or she become decisionally incapacitated.

Can I be required to have an advance directive?

No, the Federal Patient Self-Determination Act specifically prohibits health care facilities or providers from conditioning admission or provision of insurance or services upon whether or not you have executed an advance directive.

Is it advisable for me to have an advance directive, and if so, when should I execute one?

As noted above, the benefits of having an advance directive virtually always outweigh the disadvantages. Although healthy young adults may not appreciate the value of advance directives, they should appreciate the torment of the families of Karen Ann Quinlan, Nancy Beth Cruzan, and Teresa Marie Schiavo all young women who remained unconscious for the last decade of their lives. Thus, every adult, and perhaps teenagers with serious chronic illness (which frequently occasions mature thought about life, death, and the benefits and burdens of treatment), should at a minimum formulate and discuss their preferences even if they do not execute a written advance directive. And the sooner, the better.

Why do so few people have advance directives?

Many individuals do not know what an advance directive is or, if they know, they may not realize that it would be appropriate for them to have one. Many others do not have one because even thinking about the subject raises unpleasant or frightening issues. Doubtless more individuals will wish to have an advance directive when they understand how valuable it can be in protecting their right to make future health decisions for themselves and when they consider how helpful it is for their loved ones and their physician to know their preferences. This is particularly important for patients with chronic illness.

For the same reasons that everyone should have an advance directive — and for additional reasons. Dialysis is very effective in prolonging lives of those who would otherwise die of kidney failure. Fortunately, the quality of health and life for the great majority of dialysis patients is acceptable, and for many substantially better than that. Most dialysis patients are able to work and perform most of the activities they enjoy, but as many as 10% of chronic dialysis patients discontinue dialysis because they find the burdens of illness and treatment outweigh the benefits of continuing to live. Perhaps half of those who discontinue dialysis are no longer able to make decisions for themselves at the time dialysis is discontinued because of intercurrent illness with altered consciousness or because of dementia. By having an advance directive, dialysis patients are assured of having their own preferences for health-care respected, including the continuation of dialysis and of other life-sustaining treatment if that is their preference (or discontinuation, if that is their choice). Furthermore, it is a great relief to family members and to physicians to know a patient's preferences and to feel secure that they are doing what the patient would have wanted.

Why should a dialysis patient have an advance directive?

Specific reasons some individuals approaching end-stage renal failure elect not to start dialysis and reasons that patients who have been on dialysis may elect to stop it are:

Why do some people forgo or stop dialysis?

1) the presence or development of unrelated disease

which causes unrelenting pain or suffering (such as widespread cancer), extreme physical disability (such as a severe stroke or multiple amputations), or that may cause death in a very short period of time;

2) such severe dementia that the patient is unable to relate to others or to understand his or her own illness and that dialysis is necessary to sustain life (e.g., dementia from Alzheimer's disease or from multiple strokes),

3) the occurrence of such severe brain injury that the patient is permanently unconscious (e.g., from an automobile accident or following a prolonged cardiac or pulmonary arrest).

Fortunately, these various conditions with rare exception (such as a stroke in a dialysis patient whose severe hypertension is uncontrolled or such as blindness and amputations in a severe diabetic), are no more common in patients with end-stage renal disease. They do occur, however, just as they do in otherwise healthy people, and thus one should prepare for unexpected as well as foreseeable problems.

Why should a person with a transplant have an advance directive? For the same reasons that everyone should have an advance directive -- and for additional reasons. Transplant recipients other than those whose donor is an identical twin are susceptible to rejection of the transplanted organ, and thus they need to take powerful anti-rejection medications that may cause a number of complications. If the transplanted kidney is attacked by the immune system (the body's defenses against foreign substances), and if this rejection cannot be reversed, the transplant patient must return to dialysis (and thus should have an advance directive, just as all dialysis patients should). Anti-rejection medications increase the risk of infection. Serious infections may impair decision-making capacity (e.g., confusion from meningitis or delirium from any infection with high fever or low blood pressure); and if, at that time, major decisions need to be made, it would be helpful if you had an advance directive, at least one designating your preferred proxy who hopefully would know what decisions you would prefer. Transplant patients may have uncontrolled high blood pressure, and thus are somewhat more susceptible to strokes that could impair their understanding or their ability to communicate preferences (as well as cause paralysis or other serious physical impairment).

Can a teenager have an advance directive?

Although advance directives are not generally legal if made before age 21, they are certainly helpful to healthcare professionals caring for teenagers or children and helpful to parents who must make major healthcare decisions for their child. So long as the patient can understand, reason, and express his or her preferences, and so long as he or she is not depressed or under duress or coercion, statements about preferences for treatment or for a surrogate are ethically valid and should be respected

What are common errors in proxy and in treatment directives?

The most common error is naming a proxy or successor proxies but failing to inform them of your illness and possible complications and what you would wish under such circumstances. Similarly, it is a serious error not to have a three-way discussion with your proxy and your physician The next most common error in a proxy directive is naming only one individual who may not be available when needed. Another serious error is naming individuals who are not good proxies either because the emotional burden of making difficult decisions for you is overwhelming or because they are not able to effectively advocate your preferences with your physician.

Although many professionals would disagree, I believe the most common error is not having a treatment directive (relying only on a proxy directive) especially if one does not have thorough discussions with one's proxy and physician regarding one's preferences and goals. And if one does have a treatment directive, it may not be clear, relevant, sufficiently directive, or perhaps even available when it is needed. All too often directives are vague or have failed to address the circumstance that exists at the time the patient has become decisionally incapacitated. Under such circumstances, if the proxy and physician do not know the patient's goals and values which would be necessary to provide substituted judgment, they must rely on a best interests judgment which might or might not be what the individual would want.

Are there addenda that can be included in an advance directive? Yes, for example the model form in the California statute in addition to the option of designating an agent and the agent's authority and allowing for treatment preferences also provides for designation of primary physician(s), for optional nomination of a conservator (if one needs to be appointed in the future by a court), and for donation of organs at death.

There are many other matters one might wish to address in an advance directive:

1. the candor with which you wish your physician to inform you of your diagnosis, condition, prognosis, etc. or whether you wish to waive the right to be informed;

2. individuals (family, friends, caretaker, clergy) you wish to be informed of your condition by your physician and/or be consulted in making decisions for you;

3. individuals who should not be informed and who should not be consulted;

4. preferences for which primary physician, specialists (consultants, palliative care specialist), hospital, nursing home, hospice program, home health

program, etc. you wish to provide your care;

5. preference for emphasis upon goals of care (e.g., quality as opposed to duration of life) rather than emphasis on specific treatments;

6. a list of things you hope to accomplish before dying;

7. the preferred site of care when you are dying: Hospital, nursing home, hospice, home;

8. preferences for palliative care, terminal sedation, discontinuation of nutrition and hydration;

9. willingness to undergo experimental or innovative therapy for your personal benefit , or for the benefit of society even if you cannot personally benefit;

10. how literally your proxy and physician should follow your treatment directive (or how much leeway to allow them);

11. circumstances under which you would want CPR or for resuscitation not to be attempted;

12. desire for out-of-hospital DNAR;

13. the importance of preservation of your estate for your heirs (or for charities) versus expenditures for your own health care;

14. the disposition of your body or of tissues or DNA samples (e.g., for genetic testing for the information of your progeny) and whether or not an autopsy should be performed whether for the information of your family or for medical science;

15. burial or cremation;

16. organ and tissue donation or donation of one's body for research or medical education;

17. funeral or memorial service;

18. amends, reconciliations, farewells to be delivered posthumously;

19. an ethical will: statements of your values and hopes for your legacy, for your friends, humanity, and the planet.

When should an advance directive become operative?

The overwhelming majority of advance directives become operative when the patient loses decisional capacity. In California there is an option for the advance directive to become operative at once even though the patient still has decisional capacity. This option is probably rarely employed, but if the option is elected, the physician would wish to be certain that the patient does not wish to be informed (if that is the patient's desire) and/or to participate in the decision.

Where can I get help in learning about advance directives or in preparing one?

Since the Patient Self-Determination Act of 1990, healthcare professionals of all disciplines have become increasingly knowledgeable about advance directives. Virtually all hospitals, nursing homes, hospice programs, home health agencies, and prepaid health plans have written materials available for those they serve. There are many organizations such as those listed as resources at the end of this chapter which assist individuals in filling out advance directives. The National Kidney Foundation has prepared materials on advance directives to assist dialysis units and dialysis healthcare professionals as well as a brochure to educate patients (the text of which is included in this book as Chapter 14), and these are available from affiliate organizations throughout the United States.

How will anyone know I have an advance directive?

No one will know unless you tell them. You must be sure to communicate your preferences and goals to your chosen proxy (proxies), to others who are seriously concerned with your welfare and who would respect your preferences, and to your physicians. If you have written documents, you should provide your proxy (proxies), your family, your physician (s), the hospital, and — if you are on dialysis — the dialysis unit with copies, and you should take a copy with you when traveling. You should keep a list of all the individuals and institutions (and their contact information) to whom you give an advance directive.

Can advance directives be changed or rescinded?

Yes, at any time. You should reconsider your treatment preferences and update your advance directive (write a new one or change, suspend, or rescind the old one) whenever circumstances change or whenever you wish to do so. You should remember to inform your proxy, family, physician, hospital, and dialysis unit of any changes, preferably in writing. If you rescind an advance directive many recommend that you destroy all copies and the original. If you wish to change your advance directive, it is probably legal if you cross out and sign what you no longer wish and write in and sign the changes you wish, but it is probably preferable to draft a new advance directive. And if you write a new advance directive (or if you simply rescind an advance directive), I recommend that you draw a line through all outdated or rescinded copies including the original, write "rescinded" (or "replaced by a new directive on date __"), sign, and date each page. And so long as you remain decisionally capacited, you have the right to state your preferences at any time.

You cannot change an advance directive if you do not have one. If that is the case, now is the time to insure your future by executing an advance directive. If you do have an advance directive, it may already be time for you to update it!

Can advance directives be challenged legally?

Yes, in California, any interested person or friend of the patient (as well as relatives, the patient's agent or conservator or supervising healthcare provider or health care institution involved in the care the patient), has the right to petition the court to determine whether or not the patient has decisional capacity, whether an advance directive is in effect, whether planned treatment is consistent with the patient's preferences, and whether the authority of an agent remains in effect. However, the principal may indicate in his advance directive (if it is executed with the advice of a lawyer and the lawyer signs a certificate) that he does not wish a specific person or persons to have authority to petition the court.

How can I ensure my advance directive will be followed? Although there is no certainty that an advance directive will be followed and no way to ensure with certainty that it will be followed, the probability that it will be followed is substantially increased if your draft is in accordance with those preferences that your physician and agent understand and agree are appropriate. Thus, it is extremely important to discuss your goals and preferences with the agent and the physician (preferably simultaneously in a three-way meeting) and it may even be helpful to have them sign a statement that they have reviewed your advance directive and agree to honor it. It is also wise to reduce the risk of a challenge to your advance directive by discussing your preferences and goals with your family and friends as well as with all those who participate in your health care. Under all circumstances if you draft a treatment directive it should be clear, convincing, and specific especially regarding such matters as the forgoing of artificial nutrition and hydration, and especially the forgoing of oral food and fluid intake if that is your wish under certain circumstances.

Ronald B. Miller, M.D., Clinical Professor of Medicine Emeritus, founding Chief of the Renal Division and founding Director of the Program in Medical Ethics, Department of Medicine, President of the UCI Emeriti Association, University of California, Irvine.

Resources for Advance Directives

Aging with Dignity: A non-profit organization which focuses on advance care planning and publishes the "Five Wishes" document, a very popular advance directive which emphasizes personal, emotional, and spiritual as well as medical needs. The Five Wishes document "substantially meets" the legal requirements of 37 states. Even when it does not meet the state requirements, it "provides a helpful guide to family members, firends, caregivers, and doctors."
www.agingwithdignity.org   1-888-594-7437

Bet Tzedek – The House of Justice: A legal service organization in Los Angeles. Offers free California power of attorney for healthcare and healthcare instruction forms as well as information on nursing homes, residential, and kinship care.
www.bettzedek.org   1-323-939-0506

California Coalition for Compassionate Care: A statewide partnership of 50+ organizations dedicated to palliative and end-of-life care. Offers free forms in English and information in Spanish and Chinese.
www.finalchoices.org   1-916-552-7573

California Hospital Association: Offers free advance directives in English and Spanish.
www.calhealth.org   1-800-494-2001

California Medical Association: Offers a $5 advanced directive kit with extensive information, forms, and wallet cards in English and Spanish.
www.cmanet.org   1-916-444-5532
                                                          1-800-882-1262

Caring Advocates: A San-Diego non-profit organization which provides advice regarding advance care planning, consultation for proxies, and if an individual has no one he or she wishes to ask to be a proxy, it will consider serving as proxy.
www.caringadvocates.org   1-800-647-3223

Caring Connections: A division of the National Hospice and Palliative Care Organization which offers free professional advice, detailed information regarding advance care and end-of-life planning, and free state-specific advance directive documents and instructions.
www.caringinfo.org   1-800-658-8898

Center for Ethics in Health Care, Oregon Health Sciences University: Provides Physician Orders for Life-Sustaining Treatment (POLST) information and forms. These are physician orders for care and limitations thereof to cover the patient whether in the hospital, nursing home, or at home.
www.polst.org   1-503-494-3965

Center for Practical Bioethics (formerly, the Midwest Bioethics Center): A premier bioethics organization in Kansas City, Missouri which offers a workbook, called "Caring Conversations", with an advance directive document and a list of frequently asked questions. The workbook provides 47 questions (with space to write your answers) about your life, values, concerns, fears, relationships, spiritual and religious values, career, finances, legal documents and health care (which might be called a values history) to assist you in advance planning, and assist your proxy, and family in understanding and following your wishes.
www.practicalbioethics.org   1-800-344-3829

Compassion and Choices (formerly End-of-life Choices and Compassion in Dying): Offers free advance directive forms for each state with detailed explanations and with values questions that assist the principal in writing a treatment directive and assist the proxy and physician in understanding the principal's preferences. "Members receive, free of charge, counseling and guidance on how to complete and how to use advance directives. Our Client Support Program is unsurpassed in offering comprehensive service and support for individuals and families as they contemplate life's end."
www.compassionandchoices.org   1-800-247-7421

Professional Media Resources: A law firm in St. Louis which provides legally accurate and updated advance directive booklets and Forms for all 50 states for $10 (including shipping and handling), and forms in English, Spanish, and Vietnamese for California.
www.advdir.com   1-866-428-0151 (fax)

About the Authors

Rosa Adams, MSW, LCSW

Rosa Adams is a Licensed Senior Clinical Social Worker in the Department of Social Work at Olive View-UCLA Medical Center in Sylmar, California. Rosa Adams has been providing psychosocial services for children for over twenty-nine years and is a Field Instructor for the University of California, Los Angeles, School of Public Affairs and Social Work Master's Program since 1996.

Sharon Adler, MD

Sharon Adler, MD is a Nephrologist and Professor of Medicine at the David Geffen School of Medicine at the University of California, Los Angeles and the Associate Chief of the Division of Nephrology at Harbor-UCLA Medical Center. She is a member of the American Board of Internal Medicine, Nephrology Board and Associate Editor for Diabetic Nephropathy of the *Clinical Journal of the American Society of Nephrology*. She is the recipient of the Gift of Life Award from the NKF of Southern California.

Arlene Antonoff, LCSW, BCD

Arlene Antonoff, LCSW, BCD, is a nephrology social worker, divisional lead social worker for DaVita Healthcare and nephrology social worker at DaVita Tower Dialysis in Los Angeles. Active in the dialysis community for many years through her work as an executive board member of the Council of Nephrology Social Workers, she serves on the editorial board of *Dialysis and Transplantation*, volunteers with the National Kidney Foundation and is on the Medical Advisory Board of the Southern California Renal Disease Council. She participated in the original edition of *When Your Kidneys Fail* in 1982 and on its subsequent revisions.

Marilyn Appell, RN

Marilyn Appell, RN is a registered nurse with many years experience in peritoneal dialysis, beginning her career in dialysis as a hemo-dialysis nurse. She attended California State University Long Beach, California State University Los Angeles, and received her RN from Harbor College, Los Angeles. Her interests include pre-dialysis education for patients and participating in dialysis research.

Katherine Bolden, RN, MSN

Katherine Bolden is a Clinical Nurse Educator at Kaiser Los Angeles Medical Center. She is a Registered Nurse who received a Master's Degree in Nursing Education. Kathy, as she likes to be called, learned dialysis from Dr. Shinaberger at the Veteran's Administration Medical Center. It was there that she was recruited to volunteer at Kidney Camp with the NKF Southern California. She has been active with the kidney camp, recruiting nursing staff and fundraising for camp since 2000. Kathy facilitates the Regional Hemodialysis Cross-Training Course for the Kaiser Southern California Region and teaches Continuous Renal Replacement Therapy at Kaiser's LA Medical Center. She is also a guest lecturer on the renal module at Pasadena City College - R.N. Program. Kathy is very passionate about patient education and is happy to be working with the NKF Southern California on this project.

Mike Bunnapradist, MD, FACP, FASN

Suphamai (Mike) Bunnapradist, MD, MS, FASN is Associate Professor of Medicine at the David Geffen School of Medicine at UCLA and Director of Clinical Research of the Kidney Transplant Program at UCLA Medical Center. He has published more than 60 papers and presented more than 80 abstracts. He currently serves as Associate Editor for the American Journal of Kidney Disease, the official journal of National Kidney Foundation.

Nancy Chen, RD

Nancy Chen, RD, is a renal clinical consultant dietitian for Genzyme Corporation.

Adarsh Daswani, MD

Adarsh Daswani, MD was the senior clinical fellow in Nephrology at Cedars-Sinai Medical Center in Los Angeles and the Wadsworth Veterans Administration Hospital in Westwood, California, while pursuing his residency training in Internal Medicine. He has been published in *Transplantation* and *Clinical Transplants*, and his research interests include the patterns of use and outcomes of immunosuppression in kidney transplantation. His current research involves assessing the novel use of dual kidney transplants.

Susan Weil Guichard, RD, CSR

Susan Weil Guichard, RD, CSR, is a renal dietitian at the University of California, Los Angeles Medical Center for the UCLA Kidney and Pancreas Transplant Program and DaVita UCLA Dialysis Center. She was previously a clinical instructor in the Department of General Internal Medicine at the UCLA (now David Geffen) School of Medicine and coordinator for the Nutrition Section of the UCLA-GIM Residency Training Program. Ms. Guichard has authored several book chapters, including "Nutrition and the Transplant Recipient" which was published in the Handbook of Kidney Transplantation and she is a co-author of RENALTOUCH®, an interactive nutrition education system for CKD patients.

Living Well With Kidney Disease

Elaine Kamil, MD

Dr. Elaine Kamil is the Clinical Director of Pediatric Nephrology and Program Director of the Pediatric Nephrology Fellowship Program at Cedars-Sinai Medical Center, Los Angeles, California. She is a Professor of Pediatrics and serves on the Medical School Admissions Committee at the David Geffen School of Medicine at the University of California, Los Angeles. Active with the National Kidney Foundation of Southern California since she was the recipient of the Arthur Gordan Memorial Research Fellowship in 1981, she has also served the NKFSC as President, Medical Advisory Board Executive Committee and on their Board and Executive Board. She organized their first NKFSC pediatric patient education conference and continues to serve as their "kidney camp" volunteer physician. Dr. Kamil is on the Council of the American Society of Pediatric Nephrology and is a reviewer for several Pediatric, Pediatric Nephrology, and Pediatric Transplantation journals.

Mohammad Malekzadeh, MD

Dr. Malekzadeh is Professor of Pediatrics at the David Geffen School of Medicine and Chair, Department of Pediatrics at Olive View-UCLA Medical Center. He is the Director of National Kidney Foundation, Children's Kidney Camp and has been caring for children with kidney disease for over 30 years. His main areas of research interest are kidney transplantation and bone disease.

Rajnish Mehrotra, MD

Dr. Mehrotra is Associate Professor of Medicine at the David Geffen School of Medicine at the University of California, Los Angeles and is Director for Peritoneal Dialysis for the Harbor-UCLA Medical Center and the Harbor-UCLA MFI/DaVita dialysis unit. His research interests are focused in patient and physician education and his research support includes a career-development grant from the National Institutes of Health. He has published and co-authored over 50 articles and book chapters.

Disclosure of Potential Conflict of Interest:

Rajnish Mehrotra has received research support from the National Institutes of Health (NIH), Satellite Health, Shire and Genzyme Pharmaceuticals and Baxter Health Care. He serves as a consultant for Shire and Novartis Pharmaceuticals and Baxter Health Care. He has received honoraria and speaking fees from Shire and Nabi Pharmaceuticals, and Baxter Health Care.

Ronald B. Miller, MD

Ronald B. Miller, M.D. is Clinical Professor of Medicine, Emeritus and Chair of the University of California, Irvine Emeritae/i Association. After four years on the faculty at Boston University, he was the founding Chief of the Renal Division of the Department of Medicine at UCI. After receiving tenure in 1972, he was in the private practice of nephrology for 17 years with Dominick Gentile and colleagues. In 1999 he returned to the full-time faculty as founding Chief of the Program in Medical Ethics at UCI. He was a former Chairman of the Scientific Advisory Council of the National Kidney Foundation of Southern California and has particular interest in the ethics of end-stage renal disease and of stem cell research.

Ann Moore, MD

Ann Moore, MD completed her residency at Kaiser Permanente Medical Center in Los Angeles, where she is a Nephrology fellow. She has a background in molecular biology research, and is pursuing clinical research projects involving chronic kidney disease patients.

Susan Nicholas, MD, Ph.D, FASN

Dr. Nicholas is Assistant Professor of Medicine, Department of Medicine at the David Geffen School of Medicine at the University of California, Los Angeles. She is a board certified Nephrologist and holds a joint appointment in the Division of Nephrology and the Division of Endocrinology, Diabetes and Hypertension at UCLA. She is a Fellow of the American Society of Nephrology, a Hypertension Specialist and manages patients with difficult to control hypertension, diabetic nephropathy and lipid disorders. She is on the National Kidney Foundation Research Committee and is Chair of the Annual Scientific Symposium and member of the Medical Advisory Board Executive Committee of the National Kidney Foundation of Southern California.

Dechu Puliyanda, MD

Dechu Puliyanda, MD, is a Board certified pediatric nephrologist at Cedars-Sinai Medical Center in Los Angeles and serves as an Associate Professor of Pediatrics at the David Geffen Schol of Medicine at the University of California, Los Angeles. Dr. Puliyanda completed her internship and residency at Rush-Presbyterian-St. Luke's Medical Center in Chicago and her fellowship at the Children's Hospital, Harvard Medical School in Boston. Her special interest is pediatric kidney transplantation with her research focusing on viral infections in the post-transplant period and surrogate markers for renal transplant rejection. She is a member of the American Society of Transplantation, International Pediatric Transplantation Association, American Society of Nephrology, American Society of Pediatric Nephrology, International Pediatric Nephrology Association and the National Kidney Foundation.

Scott Rasgon, MD

Scott Rasgon, MD, is chief of Nephrology at the Kaiser Permanente Medical Center in Los Angeles. Dr. Rasgon ran the renal fellowship program at at Kaiser Permanente Los Angeles Medical Center from 1992 to 2005. He published articles on rehabilitation and employment in dialysis patients. His employment and education programs have won several national awards. Other interest and publications include articles on pre-dialysis care (CKD), vaccinations in the dialysis population, and sleep apnea in the CKD population. Dr. Rasgon is Chairman of the Southern California Permanente Medical Group's Annual Nephrology Symposium and is a member of the Scientific Advisory Board of the National Kidney Foundation of Southern California.

Anjay Rastogi, MD, PhD

Dr. Anjay Rastogi is on the faculty of the Division of Nephrology at the David Geffen School of Medicine at the University of California, Los Angeles. He completed his residency in Internal Medicine, his fellowship in Nephrology and his Doctor of Pharmacology at UCLA, the latter under the mentorship of Nobel Laureate, Louis Ignarro. Dr. Rastogi is also Director of UCLA's Nephrology Fellowship training program and outpatient nephrology. He heads the multidisciplinary Chronic Disease Program at UCLA and is deeply involved with Clinical Pharmacology and medical education programs.

Miroslaw J.Smogorzewski, MD, PhD

Dr. Smogorzewski is an Associate Professor of Medicine at the University of Southern California Keck's School of Medicine. He is the Associate Director of the Nephrology Fellowship Program at LAC/USC Medical Center and an Attending Physician in Kidney Transplantation Program at USC Hospital. He has been active with the National Kidney Foundation of Southern California since 1985 when he received an NKF Fellowship for two consecutive years. He has also served the NKFSC as a MABEC member, Vice President, and President; Board member; Executive Board member. His chief research and clinical interests include pathophysiology of uremia and calcium, phosphate, and parathyroid hormone metabolism, and kidney transplantation. He served as a member of KDOQI working group for Bone Metabolism and Disease in Chronic Kidney Disease.

Ashley A. Vo, PharmD

Dr. Vo is Administrative Director of the Transplant Immunotherapy Program for the Comprehensive Transplant Center, Kidney Transplant at Cedars-Sinai Medical Center in Los Angeles. She is an Associate Clinical Professor of Pediatrics at the David Geffen School of Medicine at the University of California, Los Angeles, Clinical Research Coordinator and a Heart/Lung/Kidney Transplant Pharmacist at Cedars-Sinai's Comprehensive Transplant Center. Her work has been published in journals such as *Pediatric Transplantation* and the *American Journal of Health-Systems Pharmacy* and she is currently co-principal investigator on several trials of treatment regimens for patients before and after kidney transplantation.

Judy Weintraub, MS Ed.

Ms. Weintraub holds degrees in Special Education from the University of Southern California and in Psychology from the University of California, Los Angeles. She is a former Adjunct Associate Professor at USC in the graduate program in Special Education. A patient advocate, she has lived with chronic renal failure for many years and is the recipient of numerous service awards for her work in the renal field. She serves on the editorial advisory board for *Nephrology News & Issues* and is a member of the board of directors for the National Kidney Foundation of Southern California.

Katherine Wesseling, MD

Dr. Wesseling is an Assistant Professor in the Department of Pediatrics at the David Geffen School of Medicine at the University of California, Los Angeles. Her research in renal bone disease in children is funded by the National Kidney Foundation and she cares for children with chronic kidney disease, dialyzed children, and those who have undergone kidney transplantation.

Alan H. Wilkinson, MB, BCh, FRCP

Alan H. Wilkinson, MB, BCh, FRCP is Professor of Medicine and Director of Kidney and Kidney-Pancreas Transplantation in the Department of Medicine at the David Geffen School of Medicine at the University of California, Los Angeles. A prolific researcher who has published numerous monographs, editorials, book chapters and more than 65 peer-reviewed articles in journals including *Clinical Challenges in Transplant Medicine, Transplantation*, the *Journal of the American Society of Nephrology* and *The New England Journal of Medicine*. Dr. Wilkinson is an elected Fellow of the Royal College of Physicians (FRCP), a former National Kidney Foundation Research Fellow and an hypertension specialist recognized by the American Society of Hypertension.

Index

A

F

G

H

Living Well With Kidney Disease: A Resource for Patients and Their Families

This handbook was written for the patient. We need your input for updating and revising future editions. Please help us by answering the questions below:

Which part of the handbook did you read? ❑ All ❑ Part ❑ None

Was the handbook informative? ❑ Yes ❑ Somewhat ❑ Not at all

Was the handbook easy to understand? ❑ Yes ❑ Somewhat ❑ Not at all

Will this handbook be helpful to new patients? ❑ Yes ❑ Somewhat ❑ Not at all

Did your family members read the handbook? ❑ Yes ❑ No

Are you a: ❑ Patient ❑ Family Member ❑ Other (please specify) _____

Additional comments: _____

_____

_____

_____

Thank you for your help.

Your opinion is very important to us. Please cut along dash line, place in an envelope with correct postage and mail to:

The National Kidney Foundation of Southern California
17100 Ventura Blvd., Suite 222
Encino, CA 91316-4026

Live Well!